Media Relations
for Public Safety Professionals

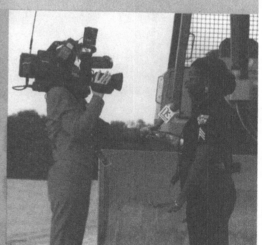

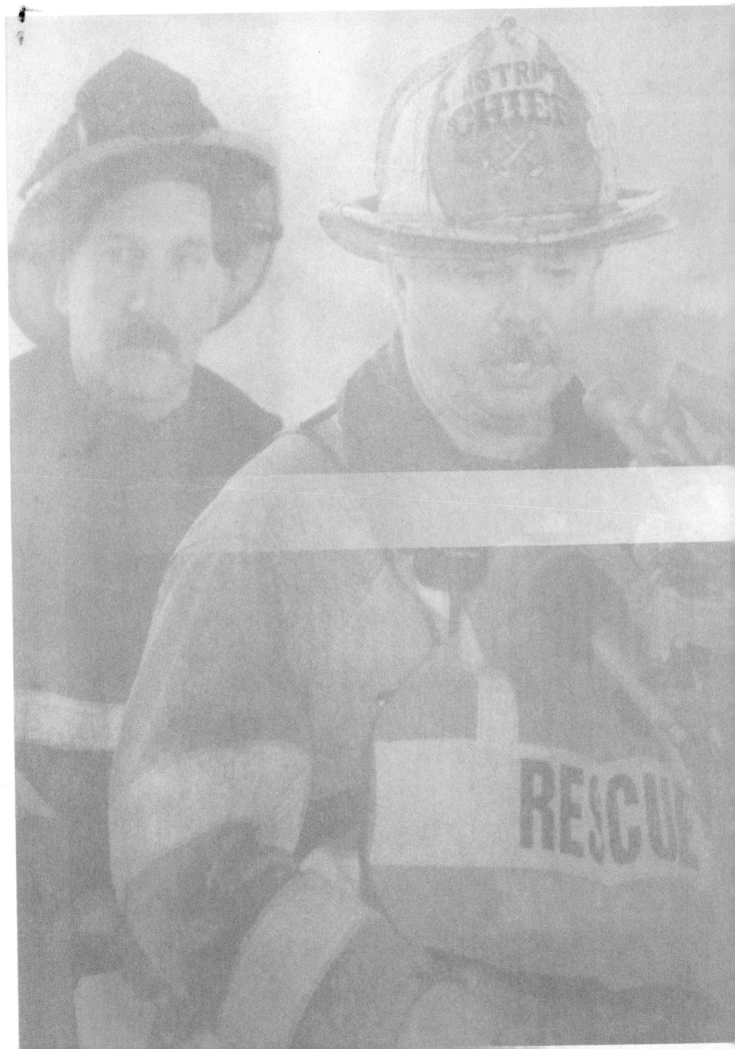

Lico M. Brown

Media Relations
for Public Safety Professionals

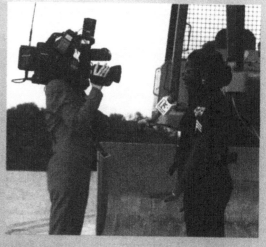

JONES AND BARTLETT PUBLISHERS
Sudbury, Massachusetts
BOSTON   TORONTO   LONDON   SINGAPORE

Jones and Bartlett Publishers

World Headquarters	*Jones and Bartlett Publishers*	*Jones and Bartlett Publishers*
40 Tall Pine Drive	*Canada*	*International*
Sudbury, MA 01776	2406 Nikanna Road	Barb House, Barb Mews
978-443-5000	Mississauga, ON L5C 2W6	London W6 7PA
info@jbpub.com	Canada	United Kingdom
www.jbpub.com		

Production Credits

Chief Executive Officer: Clayton E. Jones
Chief Operating Officer: Donald W. Jones, Jr.
President: Robert W. Holland, Jr.
V.P., Sales and Marketing: William J. Kane
V.P., Production and Design: Anne Spencer
V.P., Manufacturing and Inventory Control: Therese Bräuer
Publisher, Emergency Care: Larry Newell
Associate Managing Editor: Erin Roberts
Associate Editor: Elizabeth Petersen
Production Editor: Scarlett Stoppa
Director of Marketing: Alisha Weisman
Text Design: Anne Spencer
Cover Design: Kristin E. Ohlin
Cover Photographs (from left to right): © Julia Malakie/AP Photo; © Craig Jackson/In the Dark Photography
Typesetting: Modern Graphics
Printing and Binding: DB Hess
Cover Printer: DB Hess

The procedures and protocols in this book are based on the most current recommendations of responsible medical sources. The publisher, however, makes no guarantee as to, and assumes no responsibility for, the correctness, sufficiency, or completeness of such information or recommendations. Other or additional safety measures may be required under particular circumstances.

This textbook is solely intended as a guide to the appropriate procedures to be employed when rendering emergency care to the sick and injured. It is not intended as a statement of the standards of care required in any particular situation, because circumstances and the patient's physical condition can vary widely from one emergency to another. Nor is it intended that this textbook shall in any way advise emergency personnel concerning legal authority to perform the activities or procedures discussed. Such local determinations should be made only with the aid of legal counsel.

Library of Congress Cataloging-in-Publication Data

Brown, Leo.
  Media relations for public safety professionals / Leo Brown.
    p. ; cm.
Includes index.
  ISBN 0-7637-3167-6 (pbk. : alk. paper)
  1. Police-community relations. 2. Police and the press. 3. Police
and mass media. 4. Fire departments—Public relations. 5. Emergency
medical services—Public relations.
  [DNLM: 1. Public Relations—Problems and Exercises. 2. Safety
Management—organization & administration—Problems and Exercises. 3.
Disclosure—standards—Problems and Exercises. 4. Information
Dissemination—Problems and Exercises. 5. Interprofessional
Relations—ethics—Problems and Exercises. 6. Mass Media—Problems and
Exercises.] I. Title.
  HV7936.P8B77 2004
  659.2'93632—dc22

2003025934

Additional credits appear on page 89 which constitutes a continuation of the copyright page.

Printed in the United States of America

08 07 06 05 04   10 9 8 7 6 5 4 3 2 1

Contents

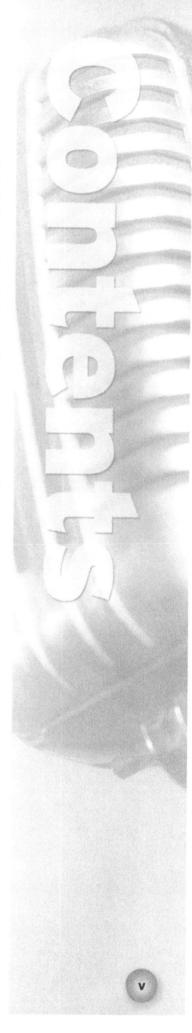

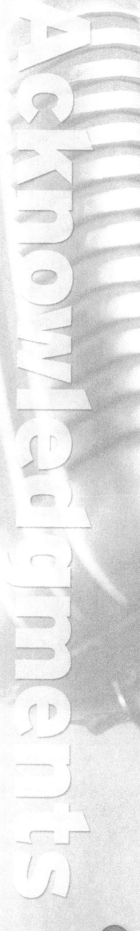

THIS BOOK WAS MADE POSSIBLE thanks to the help of some talented and caring people. My valued friend Linda Swisher, a seven-time author, supplied that all-important starting point. The following individuals provided valuable background or technical information:

Sergeant Chuck Lesaltatto, Media Liaison
Sarasota County Sheriff's Department

Agent Curtis Crawford, Public Information Officer
FBI New Agent Training

Randy Gonzales
Sarasota Technical Institute Law Enforcement Academy

Monica Yadav, News Reporter/Anchor News
Channel 40

Pat Abrams
Sarasota K-9 Search/Rescue

The knowledgeable cache of reviewers added insight and guidance:

James F. Albrecht, Captain/Commanding Officer (ret.)
New York Police Department

Andrew David

Tom Lipa, MA, CASAC
Alcohol and Drug Council of Tompkins County

Paul R. Martin, Deputy District Chief
Chicago Fire Department

Stephen P. Thomas, MS, EMT-P
AlertCPR Emergency Training

The wonderful professionals at Jones and Bartlett, including Larry Newell, Elizabeth Petersen, and Scarlett Stoppa, used their formidable skills to bring this work to the front-line public safety personnel who need it most. Finally, I thank my wife, Linda, and my children, Jarrett and Erica. Their love and support was critical during this project; without it, this book would never have become a reality.

About the Author

Leo M. Brown is a Lieutenant and public information officer with Longboat Key Fire Rescue in Longboat Key, Florida. Leo has been a paramedic for 26 years and a career fire fighter for 15 years. During his career, Leo has planned and developed Advanced Life Support Services for the Pennsylvania Department of Health; served as Affiliate Faculty at the college level for EMS training programs; authored online continuing education programs for emergency medical technicians (EMTs), paramedics, and fire fighters; and served as co-coordinator for the Sarasota County Technical Institute Fire Academy. In 2000, the Florida Association of Public Information Officers, the Florida Fire Chief's Association, and Florida's Governor Jeb Bush honored Leo by naming him Fire Service Public Information Officer of the Year. Leo holds associate degrees in Paramedic and Fire Science, numerous fire certifications, as well as a Florida adult-education teaching certificate. Leo has presented at state, regional, and national conferences for a variety of public safety personnel.

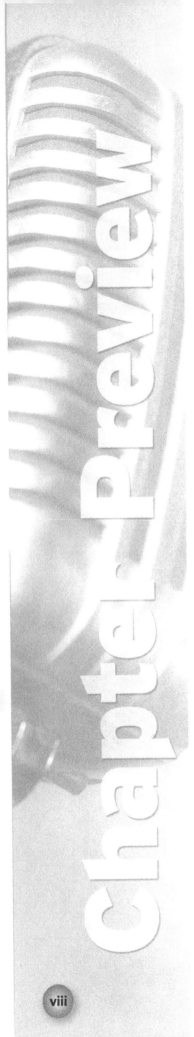

Media Relations for Public Safety Professionals is the essential training and reference tool for front-line EMS, fire, and law enforcement personnel to understand and master best practices for interacting with the news media. Whether facing a live camera at a high-profile incident or seeking to inform the community of safety concerns, this comprehensive text is designed to be a valuable resource, offering an overview of relevant laws and ethics, media policy guidelines, press releases, interviews, and more.

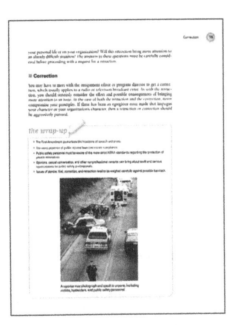

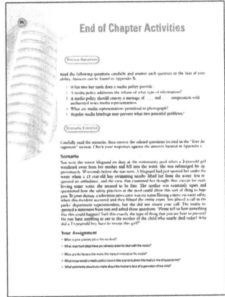

Features include:

- **The Wrap-Up** – Concise summaries of the main objectives and lessons learned from each chapter.
- **Review Questions** – End of chapter exercises to test retention.
- **Scenario Exercises** – Specific case studies and related questions to invoke critical thinking and increase understanding.

Introduction

IN TODAY'S MOBILE AND HIGHLY VOLATILE SOCIETY, the news media puts public safety professionals under constant observation. Recent national and world events, including terrorist acts, have brought the actions of emergency personnel to the forefront. Today's technologic advances allow us to gather and process information at incredible speeds. These factors have combined to make media interaction a common occurrence for front-line public safety personnel. When adding the ever-present liability issues to this mix, effective media relations training quickly becomes a top priority. Agencies must recognize this need and take steps to train in a positive and proactive manner. By providing effective media relations training to front-line personnel, organizations supply their employees with an essential tool to ensure a high level of performance.

Media Relations for Public Safety Professionals is intended to provide the knowledge and skills that are necessary for front-line emergency response personnel to deal more effectively with the media. It represents the first attempt to teach media relations from the bottom up. Previously, only upper-level officers and specially designated personnel were given instruction in effective media relations. This is no longer acceptable, as the media will often avoid speaking to the designated department spokespeople and will instead seek front-line personnel. Reporters often feel that front-line-level personnel give a more emotional response to their questions. Thus, the story becomes more valuable to the media because it becomes more emotional and gripping. As a result, media relations training for front-line personnel should be a top priority in all public safety organizations.

To date, training for front-line public safety professionals in effective media relations has been rare to nonexistent. EMS, fire, and law enforcement recruits are often instructed not to speak with the news media. Existing EMS and fire academy texts mention the subject of media relations only in passing, if it is mentioned at all. Many law enforcement academy curriculums do not include instruction on effective media relations.

Some may argue that personnel do not need this training if they do not speak to the media; however, you will learn in this text that you do not need to actually speak to the media to make a costly blunder that may then appear on the 6 o'clock news.

This book is an excellent addition to law enforcement, fire, EMS, and military training; new employee orientation; recertification/continuing education efforts; and reference materials for administrative personnel. It can also serve as a knowledge base for individuals who desire to become public information officers or for those who simply desire to be more comfortable interacting with the media.

The multiple-choice pre-test located before Chapter 1 assesses your relative knowledge of effective media relations' concepts and gives you a sample of the topic areas that are covered. The post-test, which is located in Appendix A, helps to evaluate your understanding of the course content. You should follow the chapters in sequence and complete the review questions at the end of each chapter. Also located throughout the text are scenario-based exercises, which will reinforce and measure your critical-thinking ability.

Although most examples in this book are drawn from the point of view of EMS, fire, or law enforcement personnel, they easily translate to any provider of emergency public services. Organizations such as ski patrols, lifeguards, park rangers, utility companies, transit authorities, and military personnel will benefit from the lessons provided.

The question is not if, but when you or one of your coworkers will be asked to interact with the news media. Are you ready? Do you have the necessary knowledge and skills to make this a positive experience rather than a white-knuckle disaster? If the answer is no, you now have a new and valuable tool to assist in this important aspect of your job. After completion of this text and the exercises, you should have a greater understanding of the news media and be a more prepared and professional representative of your organization.

Equipped with these valuable new skills, media interaction can now be viewed as a chance to showcase the importance of your profession and the significance of what you do.

Pre-test

Please complete this pretest before proceeding. Select the best answer for each of the following questions. After taking the exam, use the answer key to self-correct your test. Taking this short exam assesses your existing knowledge and provides a preview of the material to be covered.

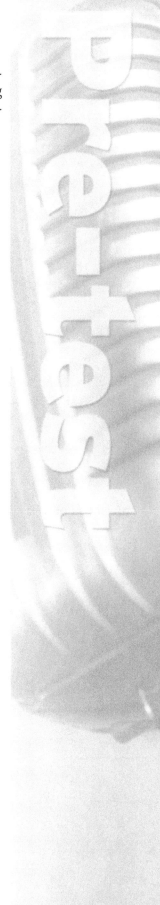

1. Which of the following individuals typically reads the news stories from the studio and is considered the chief reporter?
   a. Correspondent
   b. Beat correspondent
   c. Assignment editor
   d. Anchor
2. Which type of media relies on detailed information and does not work in real time?
   a. Television
   b. Print
   c. Radio
3. Considering the media to be the enemy is a good rule of thumb.
   a. True
   b. False
4. A beat reporter is usually assigned to cover many different areas.
   a. True
   b. False
5. The media has the same rights of access as the general public.
   a. True
   b. False
6. Libel deals with what medium?
   a. The written word
   b. The spoken word
7. According to a study, more people fear which of the following?
   a. Public speaking
   b. Death
8. A video photographer is filming a car accident in which people have been injured. What should you do?
   a. Ignore them
   b. Place your hand over the camera lens
   c. Cover the patients to protect their privacy
9. At a distance of 50 feet, you are safe from news photographers' observation.
   a. True
   b. False
10. If you are asked for your opinion at the scene of an emergency, you should do which of the following?
    a. Offer it freely
    b. Offer it with certain stipulations
    c. Offer it off the record
    d. Refuse to speculate

11. If you are asked to do an on-camera interview but are scared, what should you do?
    a. Realize that the fear will pass and do it
    b. Tell the reporter that you do not have the information that he or she seeks
    c. Inform your supervisor of your feelings
    d. Hide so that the reporter cannot find you

12. You are on the scene of a simple motor vehicle accident. A reporter asks you how many people were in the car. You should do what?
    a. Simply say "no comment"
    b. Tell the reporter that it is none of his or her business
    c. Make up a number because you are unsure anyway
    d. Give the information to the reporter

13. Which of the following would NOT be an example of a proactive media opportunity?
    a. A department promotion
    b. A meeting to discuss new disciplinary procedures
    c. Displaying new equipment
    d. Presentation of certificates to students

14. At a high-profile incident, such as a bombing, isolation of the media is the best option.
    a. True
    b. False

15. A front-line public safety provider should feel comfortable commenting on all but which of the following?
    a. Location of the incident
    b. Number of victims
    c. What you saw after arrival
    d. Estimation as to the last time the traffic light was serviced

The Media

Learning Objectives

Upon completion of this chapter, you should be able to:

- Describe how the news media operates as a business.

- List and discuss various job functions within the news media.
- Discuss different media needs.
- List the "five fundamental truths" of effective media relations.

- Define key terms that are associated with the news media.

■ How Did We Get Here?

Millions of years ago, the world was a dark and foreboding place. One day, our ancestors discovered fire. Knowing human nature, someone probably carried the fire into a cave, set someone's animal skin ablaze, and prompted an altercation. After the smoky and bleeding participants scrambled from the cave, witnesses probably traveled far and wide retelling this amazing story. This may have been the first news account of an emergency incident.

Today, except for the technologic advances, we are basically repeating history. As you exit a burning building, handcuff a suspect, or defibrillate a patient, you can count on the media being present. A major difference in today's world is the presence of microphones and cameras. Instead of your story being retold at the next cave, you can expect your voice and face to be heard and seen on every major network, as well as the Internet. This point was clearly demonstrated by the recent entrenchment of reporters during Operation Iraqi Freedom. The world witnessed unprecedented live and recorded front-line media coverage of the war in Iraq. Technology will undoubtedly continue to be the most influential factor governing the amount of media interaction we experience. The ease with which reporters can now access front-line incidents will pale in comparison to what the future holds.

This chapter should help you to understand who the news media is, what it wants, and what technology it uses. Understanding news media structure, resources, and motivation will enable you to communicate better and will make interactions (such as interviews) less frightening. This knowledge will help you to develop the skills that are necessary to make you a more professional representative of your organization.

▧ Who Is the News Media?

When trying to understand the news media, you should first remember that it is a business. Most newspapers, radio stations, and television stations are moneymaking enterprises. Some are privately held companies, whereas others are large, multinational corporations. Like any business, they must make a profit to survive, and to do this they must attract advertisers who are interested in the number of viewers they claim make use of their services. Advertising is the primary source of income for most media outlets.

Demands placed on news outlets have led to major consolidations. Large non–news-based corporations continue to acquire newspapers, as well as radio and television stations. Since these conglomerate news corporations have started slashing costs and demanding more from their media outlets, a leaner, more aggressive style of reporting has developed. Recently, relaxed Federal Communications Commission (FCC) rules regarding same-market cross-ownership has led to further consolidation by allowing a single entity to own multiple outlets within a given market.

The Internet has become the latest bone the media outlets are fighting over. This new medium has the potential to attract millions of new viewers, and this ultimately translates into a vast source of revenue. Written news accounts and video are available to anyone with Internet access. What would have been a local story in the past is now available to viewers worldwide. Large media corporations have made huge investments in the Internet in order to draw viewers and advertisers.

In an attempt to save money, some media outlets have abandoned or reduced in-house operations. Other methods to cut costs have included relying more on wire copy (news reports broadcast by large news-gathering organizations, such as Reuters, that are sometimes rebroadcast by smaller television, radio, and print markets) and the use of file footage and freelance photographers. These resources represent a significant cost savings, but can result in a less objective and more monotonous, or "cookie-cutter," style of news coverage. Only time will tell where the next great advance in newsgathering will occur, but we can rely on the fact that the business of newsgathering will become even more competitive and global in nature.

How does this information impact you as an EMT, fire fighter, or police officer at 2:00 a.m. on the scene of an emergency? It affects you in at least three ways: First, the media is being increasingly drawn to "hard" versus "soft" news in an effort to attract more viewers. You are hard news. Car accidents, fires, rescues, power failures, hostage situations, and hazardous material incidents draw readers, viewers, and therefore advertisers, who keep the news services in business. More news coverage of you and what you do means more stories, interviews, and video footage for you and your department to handle. Because the media is more often present, there is a greater chance that they will witness, record, and report on mistakes or comments that may have otherwise gone unpublicized.

If you do not have a working knowledge of the media and decide to respond to all of the media's questions with "no comment," you may have just made the day's worst decision. "No comment" is not an acceptable response, and its use only further demonstrates the need for the training of all personnel in media relations. As discussed in later chapters, "no comment" can lead the media and the public to a number of assumptions and can undermine your professionalism and credibility.

If you do not understand the role of the media, the added attention from the media to your performance makes your job more difficult. Prepare yourself for the inevitable onslaught of attention that you will face at future events by understanding the media's motivations, resources, and organizational structure.

Regardless of what many may think, the news media plays a key role in our society. News analysts, reporters, and correspondents gather information, prepare stories, and create broadcasts that inform us about local, state, national, and international events. They present points of view on current issues and report on the actions of public officials, corporate executives, special-interest groups, and others in positions of power. Some job classifications within the news industry are listed below.

Anchors introduce the news stories during radio or television programs. They also read news stories that reporters or correspondents compile. They often are linked to reporters in the field in cases in which stories are breaking as the news program goes on the air.

Beat reporters are those reporters who are assigned to cover news in one specific area (police, fire, local government, and local industry, for example). These individuals often become well known around police departments, city hall, or the EMS or fire service headquarters because of their frequent interaction. A beat reporter may also specialize in the environment, weather, society, or sports.

Commentators or **columnists** interpret the news or offer opinions to readers, viewers, or listeners. They are located in the studio but can interact with reporters in the field via satellite, microwave transmission, or even telephone.

Reporters investigate leads and news tips, look at documents, observe events at the scene, and interview people. They take notes and may also take photographs or record video footage. In the studio, they organize the material, determine and write the focus of the story, and edit any available video. Some reporters have the capability to enter information or write stories on mobile communication devices and submit them electronically from the field. Radio and television reporters often compose stories and report "live" from the scene. If time and subject matter permit, they may tape their story for a later broadcast. Newspapers, as well as radio and television stations, can require reporters to work varied hours to guarantee 24-hour news coverage.

Stringers are part-time local correspondents who work on a piecemeal basis for print or electronic media outlets.

The news business is chaotic by nature. Deadlines can leave little time to prepare a story for broadcast. Work hours must often be changed to meet a deadline or to follow late-breaking developments. Travel is often required.

Educational requirements usually consist of a bachelor's degree in journalism. To ensure a broader knowledge base, large city newspapers and radio and television stations may require candidates to have a degree in diverse subjects such as economics, political science, or business, and they often insist on a minimum of 3 to 5 years of relevant experience. Bachelor's degree programs in journalism are available at over 400 colleges or universities and include courses in mass media, basic reporting, copyediting, a history of journalism, and press law and ethics. Areas of specialization include radio and television newscasting and production, news–editorial journalism, and online newspapers or magazines.

Costly lawsuits can result from inaccurate or libelous statements. These motivators, in addition to serving the public interest, help to insure a dedication to accurate reporting.

Other valuable character traits for a career in the news business include the following: persistence, initiative, poise, resourcefulness, a good memory, physical stamina, and emotional stability. Broadcast reporters and news analysts must be at ease on camera, and all reporters must be comfortable in unfamiliar places and with a variety of people.

Reporters usually begin their careers at small publications or in small broadcast markets as general assignment reporters or copyeditors. Large publications and stations rarely hire recent graduates. New reporters are frequently assigned to cover court proceedings and civic and club meetings, summarize speeches, and write obituaries.

What Does the Media Want?

What does the media want? They are after news. They want information: depictions, explanations, and photographic accounts of what you are involved in, and they want it from you. They will ask questions, write down what is said, and photograph anything to get the information that is necessary to communicate the story effectively. The media has the right to go anywhere and take pictures of anything to which the general public would normally have access. You need to realize that this is part of our open society and in some cases is a matter of law. Specific circumstances of extreme danger or issues involving a criminal investigation can sometimes be legitimate reasons for denying media access to an incident scene or refusing to supply information.

Five Fundamental Truths of Effective Media Relations

The following five "fundamental truths" can save you much grief and anxiety when dealing with the media. Learning these simple rules can greatly help you to understand the role of the media and how to better interact with it.

Fundamental Truth #1: Your Job Is Your Primary Responsibility

Although other individuals in your department, such as the public information officer, may have media relations as their primary responsibility, your specific job should be your primary focus. Your department should maintain a policy of open but controlled communication with the media, but you must not forget your primary duty. Whether you are a fire fighter, an EMS professional, a police officer, a lifeguard, or another emergency responder, never forget or become distracted from your job. Always try to be open and professional with the media, and if time and conditions permit, supply them with the information that they need. Always remember, however, that your job is your first responsibility.

Fundamental Truth #2: The Media Has the Right to Access Certain Information

Accepting the fact that the media has the right to access certain information will make it easier for you to establish an effective relationship with the media. You should be familiar with your department's policies and with the laws of your state pertaining to your interactions with the media. Having this information will help prevent you from being caught in the uncomfortable situation of not knowing what you can or cannot say.

Fundamental Truth #3: The Media Is Not the Enemy

The "us against them" philosophy, which has dominated our relationship with the media for years, is inaccurate and counterproductive. Born out of stereotypes, television, movies, and other forms of entertainment, this philosophy persists even today within law enforcement, EMS, and fire services organizations, but it is changing. Instead, the media can be your partner in many essential activities. A few of the areas in which the news media can be a valuable ally include disseminating important information about accidents, hazardous situations, and evacuations, and reporting missing persons.

Fundamental Truth #4: Your Media Interactions Should Be Controlled

Your media interactions should be controlled. Interactions should be based on your department's media policy, your position within the organization, and your first-hand knowledge of the information requested. These three points summarize your defense plan against nervousness, apprehension, inappropriate questions, and misstatements when dealing with the media. The first point, your department policy, provides specific guidelines for dealing with the media. Learn it and use it as you would any department standard operating procedure. The second point, your position within the organization, sets limits on what statements you can appropriately make. This is important because your comments must always be "position appropriate." For example, if you are not the lead homicide investigator, you should not be commenting on leads in a particular case. The third point, your first-hand knowledge of the information, keeps you clear of the very dangerous areas of speculation and prediction. Limit your statements to what you actually saw or experienced.

Fundamental Truth #5: Never Lie to the News Media

Lying always comes back to haunt you. Your lies will show up on video, in print, or over the airwaves. You will appear foolish or discredited at best and dishonest or incompetent at the worst. The media will also often use this lie to open doors and further investigate a story that may have simply gone away had you not been dishonest.

These five simple fundamental truths can help govern your interactions with the media. Specifics for each of these concepts are presented in later chapters.

■ Important Media Relations Terminology

It is essential that you understand the terminology that is unique to media relations. A few introductory definitions are listed here to help you better understand the subject. These, together with a more complete glossary at the end of the book, will help you to better understand the news business.

- **Associated Press:** A not-for-profit news cooperative owned by 1,550 U.S. daily newspapers.
- **Criminal/investigative matters:** Examples would include arson investigations, fires involving homicide, suspected suicides, and any scene suspected to be an eventual crime scene. Requests for information regarding these matters should always be referred to the chief, the head of the department, or his or her designee.
- **Deadline:** A time limit that is imposed on the reporter before which his or her story must be presented.
- **Freelancer:** A reporter or photographer who works on a per diem basis for various news organizations.
- **Jargon:** A specialized vocabulary that is unique to a certain type of work.
- **News media:** Individuals who are directly employed by agencies of the electronic or print media.

- **News release/press release:** A prepared statement (usually written) that presents facts regarding a specific incident or event. The statement provides the "who, what, where, when, and why" of the event, in addition to a person to contact for further information.
- **Press conference:** A structured event that is held to make announcements, ask for assistance, or otherwise inform the general public about an event or issue.
- **Public information:** Information regarding policies, procedures, or events involving an organization. This may include any newsworthy information that is not legally protected, does not interfere with department operation, infringe on the rights of individuals, or endanger departmental personnel.
- **Public information officer:** An individual selected to serve as the central source of information to be released to the media and the public at large.

the wrap-up

- The news media is a business.
- The news media wants you because you, and what you do, are news.
- Today's technology can make you the top story all over the world.
- The media is not the enemy.
- Focus on your job and follow your department's media policy.

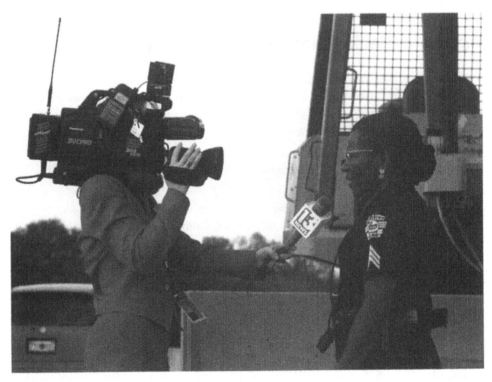

You, and what you do as a public safety provider, are news.

End of Chapter Activities

Read the following questions carefully and answer each question to the best of your ability. Correct answers can be found in Appendix B.

1. What is the most influential factor governing the amount of media news coverage that we experience?
2. What is the media's main source of income?
3. What steps has the media taken to conserve costs?
4. What important roles do the media play in our society?
5. What three factors should guide your interactions with the media?

(Scenario Exercise)

The following exercises are designed to evaluate your understanding of the material presented. They will invoke your critical-thinking abilities, enhance retention, and increase understanding of the covered topics. Carefully read the scenario, then answer the related questions located in the "Your Assignment" section. Check your responses against the answers located in Appendix C.

Scenario

You and your newly certified search-and-rescue dog, Buster, have just completed a sweep of a wooded area trying to locate Mrs. Cramer, an 82-year-old woman suffering from Alzheimer's, who wandered away from her home more than a week ago. As you emerge, a television reporter and a cameraperson approach and question you about the sudden increase in activity at the site. You and Buster have found a decomposing body. Because you are very proud of Buster's fine work, you happily tell about his outstanding performance. When asked if the body was that of the missing woman, you reply that although you cannot be certain, it may be the missing woman. Your interview is broadcast over the local news channels and is heard by all area residents, including the family of the missing woman.

Your Assignment

■ What part, if any, did emotions play in this scenario?
■ What would have been an acceptable response when asked if a body had been found?
■ What would have been an acceptable response when asked if the body was that of Mrs. Cramer?
■ What consequences could result from the speculation about the identity of the victim?
■ How might this situation have been better handled?

Learning Objectives

Upon completion of this chapter, you should be able to:

- Define ethics and discuss its impact on media activities.
- Discuss the impact of the Freedom of Information Act (FOIA) on media relations.

- Discuss the impact of the Privacy Act on media relations.
- Discuss the impact of the Health Insurance Portability and Accountability Act (HIPAA) on media relations.
- Discuss the impact of the First Amendment on media relations.
- Define libel and discuss its impact on media relations.

- Define slander and discuss its impact on media relations.
- Discuss the concept of privacy and its impact on media relations.
- Define retraction and discuss its impact on media relations.
- Define correction and discuss its impact on media relations.

■ Making a Case for the News Media

The topic of the media and the law is subject to much legal debate and would by itself require hours of study. In general, any request for agency records should be forwarded to your superior officer, supervisor, or public information officer. This chapter explores some of the laws and codes of conduct that govern media actions. Although federal laws regarding this subject will be consistent, state and local laws may differ and should be examined on a case-by-case basis. You should have at least a basic understanding of the legal and ethical justification for media actions.

Thus, a few basic but key ethical and legal points should be explored. There are laws, statutes, and codes of conduct that govern media behavior. Much of what the media relies on to justify its activities is derived from the First Amendment to the Constitution, which states the following:

Congress shall make no law . . . abridging the freedom of speech or the press.

Many court battles have been fought to either gain or deny access to certain information. Public safety personnel should concern themselves with only a few key elements of this debate. The protection of privacy should be a high priority, as this is an area where you have sound legal footing. For example, you should not release anything but the most basic information regarding individuals who are under medical care. Age, gender, and perhaps hospital destination, if known, are generally released to the media. You may not be able to restrain reporters from gathering photographs at the scene of an emergency because the media has the right to occupy and photograph any public place. You can, however, limit access to confidential patient information. Laws that protect the privacy of patient information apply not only to medical workers but also to police, fire, utility, and any other emergency responder who may have knowledge of patient information during the course of the emergency.

As explained later in this chapter, newly enacted laws, such as the Health Insurance Portability and Accountability Act (HIPAA), provide harsh penalties to those who do not protect the privacy of patient information. A generally accepted practice does allow for emergency workers to release the patient's age (if known), gender, hospital destination, and general medical condition, such as stable or serious. Name, address, phone number, specific injuries, or known medical history (such as heart attack or diabetes) should not be discussed.

At this point, you may feel a bit confused, as there are laws supporting both media access and public privacy rights. You are correct on both accounts. When the authors of the Constitution sought to guarantee freedom of speech, they also guaranteed freedom of the press under the First Amendment. This seemingly blurred line should become clearer as we explore the issue further.

■ Ethics

First, ethics and the media are not mutually exclusive terms. Although laws influence some actions of the media, professional ethics govern much of what the media does on a daily basis.

Although it is a common practice for people to identify themselves as reporters before asking questions, they may forget this practice from time to time. Our jobs would be much easier if before the interview the media was to state the following: "You should know up front that I am a member of the media and anything that you say can and will be used against you on the 6 o'clock news." Because this is unlikely to happen, you should always know the identity of those who ask questions at the scene of an emergency.

You may ask yourself whether a self-respecting, legitimate news organization would engage in unethical behavior. A survey of 304 newspapers and broadcast organizations showed that 49% of television news operations and 44% of newspapers have written codes that spell out guidelines for reporters. Most codes tend to agree on the following three principles, as defined by the Society of Professional Journalists: (1) Seek and report the truth. (2) Act independently of external pressures. (3) Minimize harm to all involved.

The National Society of Professional Journalist's Code of Ethics contains, among others, the following points:

- Informing the public is critical to democracy and justice.
- Seek truth and provide a fair and comprehensive account.
- Be honest.
- Integrity creates credibility.
- Deliberately presenting false information is never permitted.
- Seek all sides of a story.
- Identify your sources.

- Avoid stereotypes.
- Extra sensitivity is required when dealing with children and inexperienced sources.
- Realize that releasing some types of information may be harmful or discomforting.
- Remember that private people have a greater right to privacy than public or government figures.
- Avoid conflicts of interest.
- Invite public comment or grievances.
- Admit and correct your mistakes.

Although we will not discuss the entire code and its meaning, we can look at key elements of concern for public safety providers. One section of the code states that a journalist should seek and report the truth. Unfortunately, in the emergency services area, the truth is often disturbing by nature. It is not our job to shield the public from the reality of disaster or misfortune. We merely do the best we can to protect human dignity and personal privacy during the course of performing our jobs. This may be as simple as placing a blanket or other barrier to shield a patient's face. We should not, however, direct our efforts toward attempting to stop a news photographer from taking pictures of the accident.

Another section of the code addresses this topic in more detail stating that journalists should realize that certain information might cause harm or discomfort. Examples of this type of information include the following:

- Releasing of names of victims before the family is notified.
- Disclosing medical conditions or injuries.
- Releasing the names of children who are involved in any type of incident.
- Releasing graphic images without strong justification.
- Releasing inflammatory information without regard for the common good.
- Releasing information that may make the capture of a suspect more difficult or hinder an investigation.

This section of the code would seem to indicate compassion for the public; however, a few lines further in the code state that only an overriding public need can justify intrusion into anyone's privacy. When dealing with these issues, we trust the journalist's moral character to do the right thing. Sometimes this trust is justified, but sometimes it is not. We must realize that reporters, journalists, and others in the media are human beings who are susceptible to moral mistakes, errors in judgment, and character flaws. These, or any other, codes of conduct, are only as good as those who abide by them.

■ The Law

Before you become angry and begin using coarse language with the reporter who is trying to beat his or her deadline, you should know that in most cases the news media has a legal right to information. Generally speaking, the news media can go anywhere that the general public can go and has been granted access to records under specific state and federal laws, with certain exceptions. Laws granting the media access to these records vary. Consult your state regulations for specifics. The media does not, however have the right to enter private property to take photographs or gather information without permission from the owner. One of the greatest opportunities for journalistic misconduct that an emergency responder faces is speaking casually to someone who you did not know was a member of the media. This is a trap that you need to avoid. It is your job to ask—just as it is their ethical responsibility to inform you—whether they represent the media. People who are interviewed should understand that they are speaking to a member of the media and that their comments may be made public.

The media should be especially sensitive to those who are emotional or ignorant of media practices or those who do not appreciate the implications of their comments. Public safety personnel, depending on the circumstances, could clearly fall into either the emotional category or those not accustomed to dealing with the press category. Although we can never remove the emotional impact from what we do, we can become more accustomed to dealing with the press.

Freedom of Information Act (FOIA) and the Privacy Act

Most state laws governing access to information are patterned after the federal Freedom of Information Act (FOIA) and the Privacy Act. The Privacy Act (section 552a of Title 5 of the United States Code) and the FOIA (section 552 of Title 5 of the United States Code) grant certain rights with respect to agency records.

The FOIA applies to federal records within an agency, including those that are named retrievable under the protection of the Privacy Act. Any person may request copies of records under the FOIA if they have followed the required procedure as set forth under the act and the records are not subject to one of the nine exemptions.

President Johnson signed the FOIA act into law on July 4, 1966. Ten years later, Congress passed the "Government in Sunshine Act" (or Sunshine Act), which has served as a model for similar "sunshine laws" in all 50 states. The Sunshine Act was intended to make government more accessible and accountable to its citizens. Today, people on both sides of the FOIA have complaints, such as the following:

- The FOIA is an unwelcome drain on government resources.
- Lawyers sometimes abuse the act to circumvent court discovery rules (discovery refers to the pretrial devices used to obtain facts and information about the case).
- Businesses can use the act to gain an unfair advantage over competitors.
- Journalists can use the act to invade personal privacy and compromise investigations.

The FOIA has compelled federal agencies to yield millions of documents relating to government operations and performance. It seems that every week a news organization or public interest group somewhere reports information of significance to public health, safety, or good governance based on material obtained through the FOIA.

This information represents the intent of the FOIA, but the reality is something quite different. The federal government maintains millions of records. An estimated 600,000 applications are submitted each year for federal records under the FOIA. The process of applying to access these records is cumbersome and can be held up in courts for years, despite limits imposed on the government for a timely response. Difficulty in obtaining records at the state or local governmental level can vary.

The advantage for the media, and others concerned with having an open government, is that the mere presence of these laws often facilitates cooperation from governmental agencies, which have no desire to be viewed as uncooperative. Because of this spirit of cooperation, the media often receives the information that it wants. The disadvantage is that although reporters may be willing to enter lengthy court battles for records, few publishers or media executives are willing to bear the expense involved in these protracted legal challenges.

Any request that you, as a front-line public safety provider, receive should be forwarded to your supervisor or the public information officer. In most instances, it is inappropriate for front-line personnel to supply originals or copies of records.

The Privacy Act of 1974 applies to any agency records that are retrieved by name or other personal identifier and are maintained by the agency. The Privacy Act in general protects personal privacy by limiting disclosure of records without prior written consent from the subject of the record in question.

The Health Insurance Portability and Accountability Act (HIPAA) guidelines generally follow the lead of the Privacy Act of 1974. They regulate protection of patient information and require compliance (beginning April 14, 2003).

Passed by Congress in 1996, the HIPAA guidelines state that individuals or organizations that maintain or transmit health information must establish and maintain appropriate administrative, technical, and physical safeguards to insure the integrity, confidentiality, and availability of the information collected. Healthcare individuals, organizations, and other entities that come into view of another person's health information or records must provide secure access. They also require that organizations create a privacy officer to oversee the protection of these records.

Strict penalties (from $100 fine per incident for minor offenses to 10 years in jail and a $250,000 fine for major offenses) can be levied on providers who fail to comply. Federal enforcement of these regulations is carried out by the Department of Health and Human Services, the Office of Civil Rights, regional U.S. attorneys, the state attorney general, and civil litigation.

Providers can release protected health information without authorization for treatment, payment, healthcare operations, or when required by law; for public health activities; for victims of abuse, neglect, or domestic violence; for health oversight; for judicial proceedings; and for specific law enforcement activities.

Law enforcement personnel may gain access to protected medical records for a variety of reasons related to investigation, apprehension, or prosecution of those who have or may have committed a criminal offense. EMS personnel should limit the release of patient information to approximate age, gender, and general medical condition (e.g., serious or critical).

■ Libel

Libel can be defined as any written or printed matter that injures a person's reputation unjustly. If material that is written is true, it is not libel. Libel periodically becomes an issue for emergency responders. Misquotes and other inaccuracies in reporting sometimes occur. Was it libelous or simply a mistake? You and your organization must decide whether the misquote was significant enough to outweigh the often difficult process of getting a retraction or correction. Keep in mind that in addition to the retraction, you may get an even deeper probe into the incident that caused the report initially. In the case of investigative reporting, an initial story may be released to generate a complaint or a request for a retraction. This can sometimes open previously unavailable avenues for the reporter. Further complaints can work against you and can draw more attention to what may already be an embarrassing or uncomfortable situation. In cases where there has been an obvious error—whatever the cause—a complaint should be made immediately. Senior officers or representatives of the department should make these complaints, which should be directed to the supervisor of the involved reporter along with a request for an immediate correction or retraction. If the requests are not granted, you should seek legal counsel and weigh the costs and benefits of pursuing the matter further.

The other side of the libel issue must also be considered. What if you are the offending party in a case of libel? This may occur more easily than you may think. Nearly every public safety provider must prepare reports of some kind. Any opinions that may impugn an organization's character or reputation should not be included in these reports.

In the following excerpt from a run report that the responding ambulance crew filed, try to detect an example of a libelous remark:

"Medic 7 responded to a report of a choking child. After arrival, we found a 2-year-old child and mother. The mother stated that the child began choking approximately 10 minutes ago. The child exhibited no signs of respiratory distress, but the home was in a severely cluttered and unclean condition with many small objects available. This may have caused the choking incident. After completing the child's exam and clearing with medical control, we were about to leave the scene when the mother asked whether we had anything for her back pain. Considering the condition of the home, we felt sure her request was made in an attempt to satisfy a drug habit. Medic 7 did not examine the mother or supply any medication and then went available."

By committing biases in writing about the mother of the child, the crew may be guilty of libel. The crew's supposition that the mother's request for back pain medication was to satisfy a drug habit was not factual. Their own prejudices and the condition of the home influenced the crew's opinion.

■ Slander

Slander can be defined as the utterance of a falsehood that damages another's reputation. The key difference between libel and slander is the method of communication: Libel is committed via the written word and slander by the spoken word. The same caveats apply to slander regarding misquotes and requests for a retraction. The negatives often outweigh any perceived positive outcomes. You must be careful not to let your ego overrule your actions. If the impact of the story is not material and soon to be forgotten, let it go. Just as in the case of libel, you should not tolerate obvious errors. Corrections or retractions should be sought through the appropriate channels, and if needed, further legal action should be considered.

Front-line responders can also be charged with making slanderous remarks. Public safety providers involved in slander cases were frequently quoted at the scene of an incident. This quote was then recorded and rebroadcast, eventually reaching the offended party. Opinions, casual conversation, and other nonprofessional remarks can bring about swift and serious repercussions for public safety professionals. Study the following example to see whether you can identify the slanderous statement:

The lead story on the 6 o'clock news is about a traffic accident in which a congressman's son is involved. The young man had been driving too fast for the wet road conditions. He lost control and then hit two parked cars. A television news crew is rolling tape as the investigating officers are conferring at the scene. The news reporter asks one of the officers to describe what happened. This is his response: "Well, the young man was driving too fast for the wet road conditions. Witnesses stated that he was traveling at a high rate of speed when he tried to turn onto James Street and slid into those two parked cars over there."

The reporter, knowing the identity of the young man, continues, "Officer, we understand that the young man is Congressman Jeffery's son. Have you contacted the congressman?"

The officer responds, "No sir. I can't treat this case any differently just because the young man's father is a congressman. He'll be treated fairly even though that father of his never did anything for the voters, unless you count stealing our money."

The officer has broken several of the rules and thus may have slandered the congressman. He has allowed previously formed opinions to influence his statement to the reporter, and he has turned an interview into a casual conversation, thus exposing himself and his department to possible legal action if the statements are broadcast to the general public.

Privacy

Perhaps nothing, except for freedom, is taken so much for granted as our privacy. As a society, we place a high value on our privacy. Although politicians and celebrities knowingly give up much of their privacy, the general public considers it a cherished right.

Unfortunately, except for the Bill of Rights, which protects citizens against unreasonable search and seizure, no statutory privacy protection from the news media and its cameras is given. Unless you prominently display a "keep out" sign at the entry to your property, a reporter may approach and knock on your door. If this happens, you can request that they leave, and if your requests are not heeded, the reporter may be charged with trespassing.

However, once you leave your home, your right to privacy ends and you become accessible to any camera lens. A reporter may access any public place, including the scene of an accident or other emergency. He or she may also photograph and speak to anyone, including victims, bystanders, and public safety personnel.

One interesting twist is that of the semipublic place, which includes restaurants, offices, and other similar places of business. Public safety personnel often respond to these locations because they are places where people assemble. Reporters can access these occupancies but must leave if the owner makes this request. If the reporters refuse, they can be guilty of invasion of privacy but not trespassing. Legal remedies must be sought through civil court in these cases.

Retraction

Everyone makes a mistake from time to time. However, when the news media makes mistakes, the information is available for the world to see. A retraction can correct a misquote that appeared in printed material. Typically, this written statement of an error will be buried in some obscure section of the publication, as there are no rules regarding where the retraction must appear. Be warned that the media does not like retractions. To issue a retraction, the media must first admit that a mistake was made. As mentioned previously, before attempting to gain a retraction, you should look intently at the effort involved, which will probably require a meeting with the editor and other possible consequences. How valuable is your time? What was the impact, if any, on your personal life or on your organization? Will this retraction bring more attention to an already difficult situation? The answers to these questions must be carefully considered before proceeding with a request for a retraction.

Correction

You may have to meet with the assignment editor or program director to get a correction, which usually applies to a radio or television broadcast error. As with the retraction, you should seriously consider the effort and possible consequences of bringing more attention to an issue. In the case of both the retraction and the correction, never compromise your principles. If there has been an egregious error made that impugns your character or your organization's character, then a retraction or correction should be aggressively pursued.

the wrap-up

- The First Amendment guarantees the freedoms of speech and press.
- The mere presence of public access laws can create compliance.
- Public safety personnel must be aware of the more strict HIPAA standards regarding the protection of patient information.
- Opinions, casual conversation, and other nonprofessional remarks can bring about swift and serious repercussions for public safety professionals.
- Issues of slander, libel, correction, and retraction need to be weighed carefully against possible backlash.

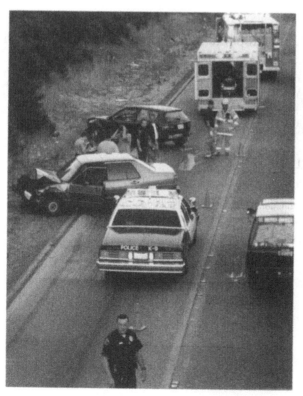

A reporter may photograph and speak to anyone, including victims, bystanders, and public safety personnel.

End of Chapter Activities

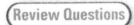

Review Questions

Read the following questions carefully and answer each question to the best of your ability. Answers can be found in Appendix B.

1. What patient information is generally released to the media?
2. Which section of the United States Constitution guarantees media rights?
3. How would you define ethics?
4. Does the media have the right to enter private property?
5. The FOIA governs what type of records?
6. The HIPAA covers what kind of information?
7. What factors should be considered before seeking a retraction?

Scenario Exercise

Carefully read the scenario, then answer the related questions located in the "Your Assignment" section. Check your responses against the answers located in Appendix C.

Scenario

You are an EMT with a metropolitan EMS service. Your supervisor has called you into her office to discuss a statement that you made to the media about the mayor's treatment for an indigestion type of pain. Your comments have fueled speculation that the mayor's health may prohibit him from finishing his term in office. The reporter in this case is considered a regular at city hall and was well known to you. Your department has no public information officer or media policy.

Your Assignment

- What comments might you have made to prompt the reporter's story?
- How and why might your comments impact city hall politics?
- What role may your prior relationship with the reporter have played in this incident?
- How might the situation have been better handled?

What Is News?

Learning Objectives

Upon completion of this chapter, you should be able to:

- Define news.
- List three types of news.
- Discuss examples of each type of news and its impact on media relations.

You Are News

News can be defined as new information, information previously unknown, or recent happenings. Thus, basically, you and what you do are news. Public safety careers naturally generate news coverage. Your function, as a public safety professional, is based on something unexpected or different occurring and your responses to these events. This chapter reviews the different types of news as they relate to your interaction with the media. This review should help you to understand what events draw media attention and why.

The Good

Although everyone likes good news, nothing attracts viewers like controversy, and good news is not controversial. As a result, it occupies a smaller portion of the news to which we are exposed. Good news does, however, have a place, and would include items such as public CPR classes, open houses, promotions, new equipment, and rescued animals. In the news business, these are sometimes called "teddy bear" stories. If you have to cut your teeth on an interview, a "good news" story is a great place to start. You are bound to say the right thing and look like a hero. Your department should make every effort to get media coverage of these types of events. The public relations value is enormous, and your agency could not afford the ink or airtime that coverage of these events would cost.

Remember to stand tall for these stories, wear your sharpest uniform and best smile, and speak with confidence. In this type of situation, everyone, including the media, wants you to look your best.

The Bad

People get into trouble, and we do our best to help them. Sometimes our efforts work out for the best, but not always. Either way, you can count on media coverage if the event is large enough. The fact that the media is present to report the news should not be unsettling. Most simple fires, auto accidents, burglaries, downed utility lines, and other mundane emergency events usually proceed without incident. Any media inquiries at these types of incidents are usually limited to time and place of incident, extent of injuries, and perhaps the dollar amount of any property damage or loss.

Remember to withhold the names of any persons, especially children, treated for injuries at such scenes. These individuals are patients and as such are entitled to privacy protection under the patient confidentiality doctrines. If you are asked about the condition of any patients, your response should be limited to age and gender of patients and the fact that they are being treated for their injuries.

The Ugly

These are some incidents from which we learn hard lessons. They remain in our memories for all of the wrong reasons. They cause the most stress to victims and rescuers alike and, unfortunately, draw the most media attention. These moments require you to be in control and stay with the facts. The "ugly" situations usually involve a loss of life, severe injury, or controversy of some type. They can often involve embarrassing or controversial situations within your own organization. Such incidents can include major fires that get out of control, arrests of department personnel, charges of misconduct, inappropriate public statements, failed rescue attempts, and many others. Emotions will be high on all sides and are part of the story in these situations. These human factors often make the ugly news the media's most covered.

These events can easily draw local, as well as national, media attention. It is not inconceivable in these situations to have media vehicles outnumber emergency vehicles. Care must be taken to not allow media coverage to interfere with emergency care efforts. Interviews should be coordinated through the EMS/fire/law enforcement media liaison or the department public information officer. The large number of people present at these events can be confusing, and your duties should not be hindered for the sake of a news report. Setting up a separate area for the media is often advisable. If informative and regular briefings are conducted at this location, the media will be less likely to wander about seeking other sources of information.

High-Profile Incidents

High-profile events include situations and issues that are not normally encountered. They can, and most times do, generate enormous public interest. Acts of terrorism have recently been added to this list. Chapter 11 specifically addresses high-profile incidents such as terrorism, mass casualty situations, and natural disasters.

the wrap-up

- Good news does not attract as many viewers as other types of news.
- Bad news is our mainstay; it is what we do.
- Ugly news is painful, but needs to be conveyed honestly.
- Terrorism has added a new dimension to the jobs of public safety providers and the news media.

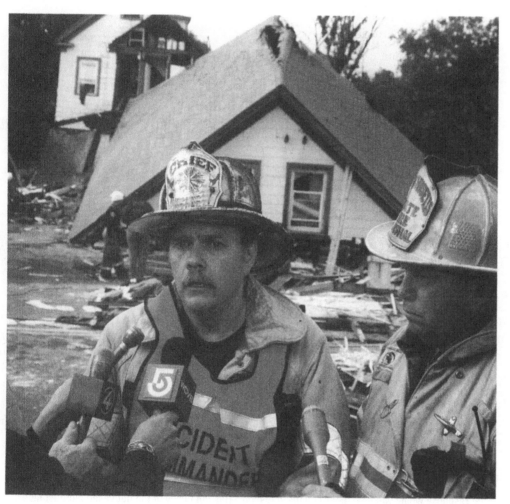

You can count on media coverage at the scene of a crime or accident. The fact that media is present to report the news should not be unsettling.

End of Chapter Activities

Read the following questions carefully and answer each question to the best of your ability. Answers can be found in Appendix B.

1. How would you define news?
2. What are some examples of "good" news stories?
3. What are some examples of "bad" news stories?
4. What are some examples of "ugly" news stories?
5. Out of the three types of news stories discussed, which one generates the most media interest and why?

Scenario Exercise

Carefully read the scenario, then answer the related questions located in the "Your Assignment" section. Check your responses against the answers located in Appendix C.

Scenario

You are an officer with a law enforcement agency that serves a community of approximately 200,000 people. After arriving at work, a crowd of reporters is outside your station. You are inundated with questions regarding the death of an uninvolved motorist who was injured during a high-speed pursuit that occurred 2 days before. Although you were not involved in the pursuit, you have been told that the motorist who was injured ran a red light at the intersection where the accident occurred. The fleeing suspect was never apprehended. Your department has a K-9 officer who also handles public information officer matters.

Your Assignment

- What response would you give regarding this question: "Has the family of the deceased motorist filed suit against the department?"
- What response would you give regarding this question: "How many high-speed pursuits have you been involved in?"
- What response would you give regarding any statements that the family of the deceased may have made?
- What response would you give to this question: "Officer, what is the policy of the department regarding high-speed pursuits?"
- What response would you give to this question: "Officer, why hasn't the department issued a statement about this?"
- Finally, how could this situation have been better handled?

The Types and Needs of the Media

Learning Objectives

Upon completion of this chapter, you should be able to:

- Define print media and list the needs that are specific to this media type.

- Define radio media and list the needs that are specific to this media type.

- Define television media and list the needs that are specific to this media type.

- Explain how the media and the Internet interact.

■ The Media's Wants, Needs, and Resources

Different types of media have different needs and ways of conveying the news; however, they all use some form of equipment to record a voice or an image. Technological advances make it possible to record voice or images over great distances. When members of the media are present, you must always assume that you are being recorded and that everything that you say or do will appear in print, on radio, or on television. This should not intimidate you, but should instead make you aware and help you to avoid an embarrassing action or regrettable remark. Today's microphones can record conversations from many feet away, and some helicopter-mounted video cameras can read the legal pad that is in your hand. Once again, always assume that you are live.

We know that the goal of the news media is to gather and communicate the news. This chapter should help you to understand the different approaches that each branch of media takes in acquiring information, which will better enable you to respond to questions and better communicate your message.

■ Print Media

The print media uses the written word to convey its message. The print media does not work in "real time." Thus, its stories are often printed hours after the event occurs and must communicate facts and emotions of the event in such a way that the reader will be able to visualize the incident without actually being present. Print media may take pictures, but written word is its primary tool. The media wants facts and details so that it can tell the story. You will often be asked for a statement and must assume that anything that you say will appear in print.

■ Radio Media

The radio media often, but not always, works in real time. Live radio feeds are possible from any location. As with the print media, the radio media relies on words—spoken words—to communicate its message. Communicating your emotions can be critical to the story. The radio media may want to talk to you and others at an emotionally vulnerable moment to add punch to the story. Assume that every microphone is live, and do not assume that because the media is comfortably behind the fire/crime scene tape that you cannot be heard. Today's microphones can record conversations over great distances. Remember, as a public figure performing a public service, anything that you say at any time can be recorded and rebroadcast. The radio media, as with all other media, will want close access to any high-profile incident. Again, remember to stay focused on your primary job while being keenly aware of the reporters' presence.

■ Television Media

Television is the most visual of all the types of media. The television media considers video (surrounded by commentary) to be the most integral part of a story. The television media communicates through images and will not only want your story, but also your face. Faces of rescuers and patients are prime targets for videographers, whose generally accepted motto is "shoot first and ask questions later." Rather than miss an opportunity, the television media will begin shooting immediately after arriving on the scene. Although television station policies differ by region and market, most have policies against showing faces of children, body bags, blood-covered bodies, or the faces of rape victims.

Today's technologically advanced video cameras can discern detail and capture sound at amazing distances. Do not assume that you are not being recorded just because a reporter is not standing in front of you. Images can be recorded from hundreds of feet away. Helicopter-mounted and mobile microwave truck-mounted cameras can record images from even greater distances. Extreme caution should be observed with all remarks from the time of dispatch until arrival back at your station or office.

Always assume that the camera is live. Reporters often want to quote you on camera. Putting a face with a story lends credibility and human interest to their report. Dealing with this type of "in your face" reporting can be intimidating. Tips to help you through this are discussed in Chapter 8. The television media, like other media, will want close access to any high-profile incident. Remember, once again, to stay focused on your primary job while being keenly aware of the media's presence.

■ Internet Media

After the USSR's launch of Sputnik in 1957, the United States Military, led by the Department of Defense, began a race to establish a leadership position in the area of science technology. These efforts had early and significant contributions to the creation of the Internet. The sharing of information over distances eventually led to the concept of connecting remote computers. This gave rise to the creation of the first e-mail program in 1972. With the coining of the term Internet in 1974, the United States Military and various academic institutions combined to make rapid advances leading to the World Wide Web and the global exchange of information that we now enjoy.

Whether by design or necessity, the media has become a major user of the Internet. All major news services have Internet sites where users can access online versions of their news. Areas of the world that previously had no, or only local, radio or television outlets are now connected to the entire world via these Internet news services.

A full-color image of you arguing with a photographer at the scene of an incident can now be seen by anyone in the world with access to the Internet. These stories can now be accessed via cell phones, PDAs, or pagers. When it comes to newsgathering, you no longer live in Small Town, USA; you live in the world, via the World Wide Web. Your successes and failures have the potential to be broadcast worldwide. The up side of this situation can be just as dramatic. The resources that are available to you and your organization have expanded exponentially. You can access research that was previously unavailable or difficult to obtain. Disaster plans, treatment protocols, and news reports are all at your fingertips. You can also share your information and experience with the public safety community. The Internet is an incredibly rapid, vast, and easily accessible resource for both you and the media.

the wrap-up

- When the media is present, you must always assume that you are being recorded and that everything you say or do will appear in print, on radio, or on television.
- The print media may take pictures, but the written word is their primary tool.
- The radio media relies on spoken words to communicate their message.
- The television media often thinks that the video (simply surrounded by commentary) is the story.
- Public safety personnel and the media can use the Internet as a resource.

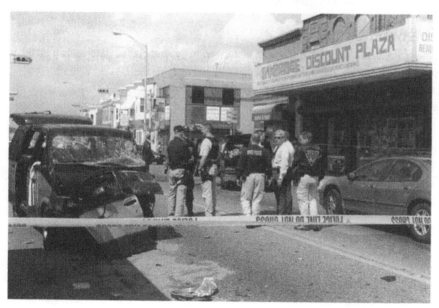

Assume you are being recorded even when the media are stationed a far distance from the scene.

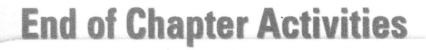

End of Chapter Activities

Review Questions

Read the following questions carefully and answer each question to the best of your ability. Answers can be found in Appendix B.

1. Which type of media relies most heavily on the written word?
2. How important is video to the television media?
3. At what distance are you safe from the media cameras?
4. What assumptions should you make when microphones and cameras are present?

Scenario Exercise

Carefully read the scenario, then answer the related questions located in the "Your Assignment" section. Check your responses against the answers located in Appendix C.

Scenario

You have just finished reading a reporter's story about an automobile accident at which you were assigned traffic control. This particular intersection has been the scene of numerous accidents because of the lack of a traffic control light. You were interviewed at the scene, and the reporter prefaces your quote by saying, "When interviewed at the scene, even law enforcement personnel thought that it was negligent of city officials to delay putting in a traffic control light at this intersection."

Your Assignment

- What comments might you have made during this interview to generate these statements from the media? If you choose, you may take the position that you were misquoted. If so, explain your options.
- How might your alleged comments impact public opinion on this issue?
- How might the situation have been better handled?

Create a Policy for Dealing With the Media and Follow It

Learning Objectives

Upon completion of this chapter, you should be able to:

- Identify the purpose of a media policy.

- List the components of a media policy.

- Define local media.

- Define national media.

- Discuss methods to deal with national versus local media.

- List common components of a press release.

■ Why Have a Media Policy?

Just as the standard operating procedures and recommended operating guidelines provide guidance in other aspects of your job, a media policy provides two key tools to assist you in communicating with the media: direction and performance objectives. These tools will help you to make critical decisions at times of great stress. With the increase in media exposure that we are all sure to encounter, it would seem negligent not to have a policy that guides our interactions with the news media. This chapter explains the components of a media policy, local versus national media, and the press release. Although an in-depth discussion of how to develop and implement a media policy is beyond the scope of this text, several aspects of the policy itself can be discussed. Included are excerpts from a sample media policy.

The purpose of a departmental media policy is to provide guidelines for the release of public information to print and electronic news media.

The policy should be written so that it conveys a message of full and impartial cooperation with authorized news media representatives in support of their efforts to gather public information pertaining to the activities of your organization. The policy should state that these efforts should not interfere with departmental operation, infringe on individual rights, or violate any law.

■ The Components of a Media Policy

A successful media policy contains several key components. The following information is not intended to represent a complete media policy but rather to demonstrate areas that would apply to front-line public safety personnel on a daily operational basis.

Purpose

The purpose section within a media policy outlines the intent of the policy, essentially why it exists. An example of a media policy's purpose may be written as follows:

PURPOSE: To set forth uniform guidelines for the release of information and to establish responsibilities of the public information officers and other department personnel in dealing with the media.

It should be noted that all personnel are public information officers for the department, but each person has a different level of responsibility. As such, all personnel should cooperate with the media to the extent that their knowledge and authority permit. If, at any time, questions should arise about how to proceed, personnel should seek the advice of their immediate superior or the public information officer.

Policy Statement

The policy statement within a media policy provides the governing principles by which a public safety organization abides in their interactions with the media. A policy statement may be outlined as follows:

POLICY: It is the policy of the _____ Fire/Rescue/Police Department to cooperate with the media whenever possible within the guidelines of the State of _____ public records law and the procedures contained in this guideline. It will be a matter of policy for the department to communicate information to the fullest extent without compromising investigations or public safety.

Authority, Responsibility, and General Guidelines

Other key components that may be covered in a successful media policy include (1) authority and responsibility, (2) on-scene authority, and (3) general guidelines. Examples of written policies are listed below:

AUTHORITY AND RESPONSIBILITY: The EMS/police/fire chief has the authority and responsibility to maintain an on-call public information officer for all major incidents. The public information officer is responsible for training and maintaining a list of all qualified members of the department for possible public information officer duties.

ON-SCENE AUTHORITY: The fire investigator, police supervisor, senior fire officer on scene, or their designee shall be the department spokesperson in the absence of the public information officer.

GENERAL GUIDELINES: All personnel are encouraged to cooperate with the media as much as possible. Personnel who speak to the media should limit the information to response actions taken after their arrival and to any first-hand knowledge. When you cannot accommodate media requests for information, efforts should be made to be as courteous as possible. Personnel shall not release medical information that would represent an invasion of privacy, or information that may compromise any investigation. Names of any person under medical care or deceased shall not be released. Personal opinions should never be expressed to any media representative. Be advised that anything you say is public record.

Media Access

As mentioned in Chapter 3, the media has a right to be present at an emergency scene, but care must be taken to not allow media coverage to interfere with emergency care efforts. The following media access policy serves to protect the public safety personnel, the media, and the public:

MEDIA ACCESS: Although our first priority is to respond appropriately to emergency situations, personnel should extend courtesy to the media at emergency scenes. Media vehicles and equipment should be permitted closer access to the incident than the general public without obstructing operations. Use of barricade tape should be used to mark clearly the perimeters for public and media access. If requested, media representatives shall be directed to the media area, the public information officer, or their designee. Personnel shall not obstruct the media in the performance of their duties unless personal injury is imminent or operations will be impeded. Personnel should never physically block camera shots or touch media equipment, except as previously indicated. Personnel shall neither discourage nor encourage the media in photographing or televising anything within their view. As a general rule, the media may photograph anything in public view.

Public Information Officer

Public information officers have media relations as their first responsibility. As defined in Chapter 1, the public information officer is an individual selected to serve as the central source of information to be released to the media and the public at large. Taking into consideration this individual's responsibilities, it is important that your organization's media policy include a section regarding this role. See below for an example of a good public information officer policy:

PUBLIC INFORMATION OFFICER: The public information officer or on-call designee shall respond to all incidents as warranted and report to the incident commander and shall be automatically paged/phoned or otherwise notified of all major incidents, working fires, officer-involved shootings, severe injuries, or deaths of department personnel. The public information officer or designee shall work with responding law enforcement agencies if necessary to establish a media area inside the perimeter that is established for the general public. This area should be selected to enable the media to obtain photographs and videos of the event while ensuring its relative safety and noninterference with the operation. The location should be near the command post, but out of normal speaking voice range if possible. The public information officer or designee shall work closely with the incident commander in gathering information and determining what shall be released pursuant to legal guidelines and departmental policy. The public information officer or designee shall establish and maintain a liaison with all on-scene media representatives and assist them with their news-gathering efforts, while ensuring noninterference with departmental operations and preserving the integrity of any investigations. The public information officer or designee shall provide periodic briefings to the media and, if conditions allow, should encourage the incident commander and/or another member of the department involved in newsworthy activities to be available for interviews. Two problems that can be prevented by regular briefings are freelancing and speculation. At the conclusion of the incident, the public information officer or designee may prepare and disseminate a news release that documents the event for local news organizations. In cases involving sensitive matters or continuing investigations, the public information officer or designee shall review the release with the incident commander or investigators before release.

Local Versus National Media Coverage

Most of your interactions with the media will be with individuals from your local media market. As you build a working relationship with them, you will begin to understand and trust each other, which will lead to a smooth and effective flow of information and effective communication in times of crisis.

At some time, however, you may draw the attention of the national news media. Out-of-town reporters and satellite relay trucks from large market and wire news services will inundate your community. The ensuing chaos can often lead to a shunning of the local media in favor of the large, national news services. You can avoid making this mistake by remembering to treat everyone equally and fairly. Information should be made available to all media outlets, with no favoritism. The large media outlets will disappear soon after the event is over, perhaps never to be seen again. However, if the local media was shunned or preferential treatment was given to the national networks, your relationships with the local media could suffer. If this occurs, do not expect coverage of your next open house or training event.

The reverse is also true. If you favor the local media, you may not get the extensive coverage necessary to pass along vital information about the incident, and you may be initiating a problem such as the one described in the Scenario Exercise at the end of Chapter 2, in which a reporter and a public safety worker become friends.

Generally, during large-scale events, department public information officers or senior officers will have control of the situation and will ensure equitable distribution of information; however, all personnel should be aware of this potential problem so that any conflicts are avoided.

The Press Release

A front-line public safety provider would not normally write a press release. However, you may be the subject of a press release. Press releases serve many useful purposes, including:

- Notifying the media of public relations events, such as open houses.
- Announcing public education events.
- Providing notice of public health or safety issues.
- Providing notice of hazardous weather conditions.
- Making requests to locate missing or sought after individuals.
- Providing notice of significant interdepartmental events, both positive and negative.

Following, the key components of the press release are briefly covered. These give you insight into the mindset of assignment editors, whose job it is to select which events deserve news coverage. First, consider this: The primary purpose of the press release is to inform others about a recent news event. Old information has little or no value to the media. Thus, a press release must be timely so that the media will take an interest in what you have to say, and so that your information will have a better chance of being printed or aired. Putting information into writing leaves less room for misinterpretation. You may head off speculation by making this preemptive move. What you put in the release may be enough to keep the media at bay until you can gather more information. Although the media can, and in most cases will, seek out other sources of information, issuing the release helps you to portray your side of the story and thus balance the account of the incident.

Writing a poor press release is probably the best way to ensure that the media will ignore your story. Assignment editors are very busy people. If their attention has not been grabbed in the first few sentences, forget it: You and your story will quickly be passed over. The following are key components of the press release, with rationale for each:

- **For immediate release:** If your story is not for immediate release, it probably is not newsworthy.
- **Name and address of your organization:** Place this in bold type, as it may determine whether the editor reads any further.
- **The topic or headline:** This tells the editor where he or she should direct the release; it should be an attention grabber.
- **Paragraphs:** The most important information should be listed first. The editor's attention needs to be grabbed in the first few sentences.
- **Name of author and contact information:** This is essential. You may have a great news story, but if the editor does not know who to contact or if the information is incorrect, the information will not be used.
- **"More" or "###" at the bottom of the page:** "More" tells the editor that there are more pages, and "###" signifies that he or she has reached the end of the release. Press releases should never be more than two pages (one page is preferable).

These tips should help you to understand what drives the news media and how errors in the preparation of a press release affect your chances of obtaining media coverage.

the wrap-up

- A media policy provides instructions and baseline performance objectives for communicating with the media.
- The policy should be written so that it conveys a message of full and impartial cooperation.
- Personnel shall not release medical information (which would represent an invasion of privacy) or investigative information (which may compromise an investigation).
- Personnel shall not obstruct the media in the performance of duties unless personal injury is imminent or operations will be impeded.
- Press releases should be timely and accurate.

End of Chapter Activities

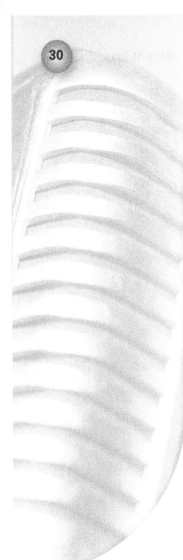

Review Questions

Read the following questions carefully and answer each question to the best of your ability. Answers can be found in Appendix B.

1. What two key tools does a media policy provide?
2. A media policy addresses the release of what type of information?
3. A media policy should convey a message of ____ and ____ cooperation with authorized news media representatives.
4. What are media representatives permitted to photograph?
5. Regular media briefings may prevent what two potential problems?

Scenario Exercise

Carefully read the scenario, then answer the related questions located in the "Your Assignment" section. Check your responses against the answers located in Appendix C.

Scenario

You were the senior lifeguard on duty at the community pool when a 2-year-old girl wandered away from her mother and fell into the water. She was submerged for approximately 30 seconds before she was seen. A lifeguard had just spotted her under the water when a 15-year-old boy swimming nearby lifted her from the water. You requested an ambulance, and the crew that examined her thought that, except for swallowing some water, she seemed to be fine. The mother was extremely upset and questioned how the safety practices at the pool could allow this sort of thing to happen. To your dismay, a television news crew was on scene filming a story on water safety when this incident occurred and they filmed the entire event. You placed a call to the parks' department superintendent, but she did not return your call. The media requested a statement from you and asked these questions: "Please tell us how something like this could happen? Isn't this exactly the type of thing that you are here to prevent? Do you have anything to say to the mother of the child who nearly died today? Why did a 15-year-old boy have to rescue this girl?"

Your Assignment

- What is your primary job in this incident?
- What important steps have you already taken to deal with the media?
- What are the factors that make this story of interest to the media?
- What value would a media policy have in this scenario given the media's line of questioning?
- What comments should you make about the mother's lack of supervision of the child?

Why "No Comment" Is an Unacceptable Response

Upon completion of this chapter, you should be able to:

- Explain how television and other entertainment outlets have influenced the attitudes of law enforcement, EMS, and fire department personnel toward the media.

- Explain how "no comment" affects your side of the story.

- Explain the link between "no comment" and suspicion.

- Explain the link between "no comment" and assumptions about your ability or desire to answer questions.

- Supply possible alternatives to the "no comment" response.

■ How the Past Has Shaped the Present

"No comment." We have all heard it, read it, and seen it a hundred times. However, "no comment" is not an acceptable response to questions from the media, and such a response can potentially create a number of avoidable problems. Every emergency responder, no matter his or her rank or position, should feel confident in his or her ability to communicate calmly and professionally with the news media. Departments with a "no comment" policy are engaging in an unproductive exercise that will serve only to alienate the media and the public.

Although it is true that good news is better than bad news, even bad news is, on occasion, better than no news. No news, more frequently expressed as "no comment," is often greeted with suspicion or mistrust and serves to undermine the confidence of the media and the community in your department. This chapter explains how adopting an open but controlled policy of dealing with the media allows your department to take advantage of the many benefits of fast and effective communication, while still maintaining the necessary control over privacy and legal issues.

You need to remember this: If you do not give the media information, they will simply ask someone else, who may not be qualified to provide information about the event. The following are questions you should ask yourself about potential situations that may arise if you choose not to provide information:

- Would you rather that the media receive the facts from one of your informed representatives, or from the neighbor who just came home from a night on the town but swears that it took you over 30 minutes to arrive on the scene?

- Would you rather that the media receive an account of the situation from your incident commander, or from the gentleman on the scene who has been left homeless by arson in the last year?
- Would you rather that the media hear from your representative, or the brother of the defeated mayoral candidate who based his campaign on police department cutbacks?

Having a representative from your organization explain the details of an incident in a calm and professional manner is a more intelligent and appropriate option. Your representative speaking to the media will not preclude reporters from seeking other sources. It will, however, allow your side of the story to be told and therefore provide balance to whatever news report should result.

Are You Hiding Something?

When confronted with the "no comment" phrase, human nature leads us to suspect that someone is hiding something. "No comment" conjures up images of alleged criminals seated in a courtroom. Gang leaders, mob leaders, and corporate leaders alike cling to the phrase as their protection from prosecution and penalty. Why would an innocent person refuse to speak? Who is he or she trying to protect? What terrible deed is he or she concealing? These and many more questions arise in the public's minds when the phrase "no comment" is heard.

This suspicion is especially true in high-profile incidents that involve injury or death. The mere appearance of a cover-up or concealment of information will heighten public interest and drive the media elsewhere for the answers that they need. The media will often begin their next interview with your statement of "no comment," using it as a springboard for questions. For example, the media may seek your supervisor or another official and ask the following question: "Chief Williams, we just spoke with Lieutenant Smith at the scene of the building collapse that injured two fire fighters. His only response to our questions was 'no comment.' Chief, how could the officer at the scene of an accident like this have nothing to say? Didn't he know the dangers involved? Chief, is the department hiding something?"

As you can see from this example, "no comment" can open doors leading to inappropriate lines of questioning. Even in cases in which all of the information is not yet available, an officer can take a moment to give a cursory explanation of what has happened. This may redirect the reporter's thought process, and he or she may take a different approach to the situation.

Are You Uninformed?

If you are going to make a statement to the press, you must be a credible source. "No comment" leads the reporter and the general public to make assumptions. You are either hiding something or are not the person to talk to because you simply do not know what is going on. If your comments make it to the airwaves or a television news report, you and your department can look unprofessional and uninformed.

Assumptions may be made and comparisons drawn between your apparent failure to have information at hand and any unfortunate events that may have occurred at the incident. As in the previous example, refusing to comment may lead to speculation that you do not know what is going on around you. If you are a front-line public safety provider, you may have limited knowledge about an incident at a major disaster. In this case, a "no comment" response is an unnecessary attempt to protect or shelter information that you are not expected to possess. Simply stating that you do not know is much more prudent.

On the other hand, if you are a senior officer or incident commander at the scene, a "no comment" response can be interpreted more harshly, as you are expected to know and be in control. These are all legitimate expectations under normal circumstances. As we all know, emergency incidents are anything but normal, and the media is aware of this fact. Still, you should make every effort to provide up-to-date and factual information. If you cannot provide information at the time but may be able to at a later time, then say so. Avoid the "no comment" response to maintain your credibility.

Are You Being Uncooperative?

Another assumption that can result from a "no comment" reply is that if you are not hiding something and you do have the information, then you are simply being uncooperative. This is, in some people's minds, the next logical conclusion when the other possibilities have been eliminated. At the level of front-line personnel, many reasons for not providing the requested information exist. You may want to cooperate, but are inhibited for one or more legitimate reasons that have nothing to do with a cover-up or vendetta against the news media. The reality may simply be that you are not commenting for one or more of the following reasons:

- You are afraid or uncomfortable with the entire interview process.
- You may not have the skills that are necessary to participate.
- You may not want to be the center of attention.
- You may not want to say the "wrong thing."
- You may have had a bad experience with the media in the past.

These and many other reasons may seem quite rational in your mind; nevertheless, people will always assume the worst when they hear "no comment." Some of us, because of the rough-and-tough image associated with what we do, could never imagine stating this to the reporter: "I really feel uncomfortable in front of a camera and would rather not be interviewed." Our own words would make us feel embarrassed and belittled. How could we chase the fleeing armed robbery suspect, run into the burning building, or dive into the pounding surf without hesitation and then be afraid of a television camera or a microphone? There is nothing wrong with admitting your fears and explaining your reasons for not wanting to make a statement. This type of response is very unlikely to be interpreted as being uncooperative. In fact, it can send a very positive message to your community. It tells them that you are human. The cumulative effect of this type of good press is invaluable over time. From a public relations point of view, this unrehearsed, unplanned imagery of a public safety provider being human is invaluable.

Alternatives to the "No Comment" Response

If you cannot say "no comment," what can you say? Although this question is addressed more thoroughly in Chapter 8, a few appropriate alternatives to "no comment" include the following:

- I do not have that information but can refer you to someone who may be able to help.
- The investigation is being conducted at this time, and we cannot comment until all of the facts are available (please note that "cannot comment" is significantly different from "no comment").
- The situation is still evolving, but we will be issuing a statement as soon as possible.

All of these responses, and many more, are dependent on the situation. The key points to remember are as follows:

- When in doubt, refer to someone else who can be of assistance.
- Do not guess.
- Do not lie.
- Do not be afraid to say that you do not know.

the wrap-up

- Departments with a "no comment" policy are engaging in an unproductive exercise that will only serve to alienate the press and the public.
- Adopting an open, but controlled, policy of dealing with the media allows your department to take advantage of the many benefits of fast and effective communication, while still maintaining the necessary control over privacy and legal issues.
- When confronted with the "no comment" phrase, human nature leads us to suspect that someone is hiding something.

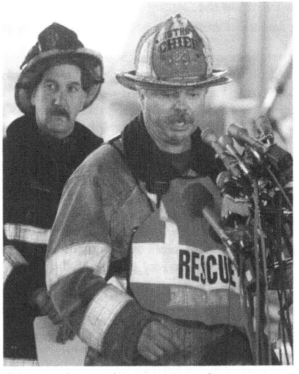

If you are going to make a statement to the press, you must be a credible source.

End of Chapter Activities

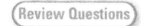

Read the following questions carefully and answer each question to the best of your ability. Answers can be found in Appendix B.

1. What two groups do a department that adopts a "no comment" policy alienate?
2. What are two benefits of having your department spokesperson tell your side of the story?
3. What negative image is invoked by the phrase "no comment"?
4. What are acceptable alternatives to saying "no comment"?
5. What are some legitimate reasons for not wanting to participate in an interview?

Scenario Exercise

Carefully read the scenario, then answer the related questions located in the "Your Assignment" section. Check your responses against the answers located in Appendix C.

Scenario

The fire chief has just requested that you report to his office immediately. His concern is regarding a fire that you and your crew fought several hours ago. As the station lieutenant, you served as the incident commander for the first 10 minutes of the fire. The property owner has already placed calls to the mayor, the fire chief, and the media to refute a news story in which you were quoted as saying that the fire had to be arson because the building had been unoccupied for so long.

Your Assignment

- Were your comments appropriate or inappropriate given your role at the incident? Defend your answer.
- What legal complications may result from your alleged comments?
- How might the situation have been better handled?

7 Public Speaking and Its Associated Problems

Learning Objectives

Upon completion of this chapter, you should be able to:

- Define social phobia.
- Define specific phobia.

- List phobias that are associated with public speaking.
- Explain why a reporter does not want you to be too "polished."

- List techniques to lessen tension during an interview.
- Explain how changes in the reporter's line of questioning can affect the interview.

■ Not Everyone Wants to Be in the Limelight

If you are like most people, you probably dread speaking in public. However, you possess more than the required amount of skill to overcome your apprehensions. Like most of us, you may have a few butterflies. This chapter identifies causes and suggests methods for overcoming fears of public speaking. Some of these causes have deep psychological roots, whereas others are simply the fear of something new. In either case, suggestions are discussed for dealing with these fears in an effort to make you as comfortable and professional as possible when speaking in public.

■ Phobias

In extreme cases, individuals may actually suffer from a medically diagnosed phobia of public speaking. According to the National Institute of Mental Health, a social phobia, also called a social anxiety disorder, is a disorder characterized by overwhelming anxiety and excessive self-consciousness in everyday social situations.[1] People with a social phobia can, among other things, have a fear of being watched, judged, or humiliated. Any of these fears can be associated with public speaking or participating in a media interview. Social phobia affects approximately 5.3 million adult Americans.[2] The National Institute of Mental Health describes a specific phobia as an intense fear of something that poses little or no actual danger. Phobias often represent an irrational fear that people may or may not be able to avoid in their daily lives. Specific phobias affect an estimated 6.3 million adult Americans.[1] Someone with a fear of any type of media contact should be allowed to avoid the situation and should never be forced to participate.

Although the majority of people simply suffer from a case of the jitters, those individuals who exhibit extreme fear of speaking in public should never be forced to do so. Placing someone in this position is a no-win situation and will not best serve your department or the public. If you are asked to participate in an interview and do not feel comfortable doing so, inform your supervisor immediately.

Phobias Associated With Public Speaking

If you have, or feel that you may have, any of the following conditions, avoid public speaking without first seeking the help of a professional therapist.

- **Glossophobia:** Fear of speaking in public. This may exclude any public safety provider from participating in an interview.
- **Opthalmophobia:** The fear of being stared at. If you feel uncomfortable speaking in front of a small group, speaking into a camera, which represents thousands of eyes, may be terrifying.
- **Atychiphobia:** The fear of failure. This can affect individuals who are suddenly placed in the limelight. If you have little or no training and no time to prepare your response, fear of failure can be a powerfully negative influence on your emotions.

The Media Does Not Want Perfection, They Want You!

Assuming you do not have a medically diagnosed phobia; instead, you may have a huge case of butterflies, nerves, jitters, stage fright, or whatever name you choose. However you label it, you are afraid. You may fear making a mistake, looking foolish, saying the wrong thing, or freezing and thus, saying nothing at all.

Remember that you are not expected to be an expert in broadcasting. In fact, that is why you were selected for an interview. The media does not necessarily want a smooth, polished, public relations professional. It wants the soot-stained, sweaty fire fighter who just exited the burning building carrying a rescued child. It wants the police officer who just chased and captured the fleeing suspect. It wants the utility worker who just emerged from the drainage pipe holding the kitten. It wants the search and rescue team emerging from the forest carrying the lost young child. It wants the lifeguard emerging from the water after saving the exhausted swimmer.

Tension Busters

A few tricks are available for you to combat the inevitable nervousness. First, take a deep breath. Whether a print, television, or radio reporter is interviewing you, a few relaxation techniques can help you to combat nervousness.

Unfortunately, the best technique for combating fear of public speaking is practice. Although few of us have this option, all is not lost. One technique that is surprisingly effective in reducing fear is to admit to the reporter and to yourself that you are nervous. This simple act breaks down the wall between yourself and the reporter and makes the interview more of a conversation than an inquisition.

Releasing excess physical energy that stress causes can be helpful. Try tensing and relaxing your fists or other parts of your body a few times. If possible, do this out of camera shot and keep your hands at your sides; otherwise, you may look like someone who is preparing for a fight rather than for an interview. Take a breath each time that you tense. Exhale each time that you release. Close your eyes while you do this, if necessary. Focus on moving the air in and out of your body. Numerous other techniques exist, but choose wisely, as you do not want the lead story on the 6 o'clock news to be footage of you jogging in place while singing the national anthem.

Another option that has proven to be very effective is the "buddy interview." You can ask that an associate be present and interviewed with you. This tag-team approach is popular with the television media, as it puts more faces on camera. The media can use the support and camaraderie between you and your partner as another angle for the story. It is amazing how this simple technique can reduce tension. However, if the time slot for your story is limited, do not be surprised if the second person is edited out at the studio. If this occurs, be thankful that your "buddy" was present and supported you during the interview.

If none of these techniques work, try forgetting about the microphone or camera. The equipment is often the source of people's jitters. Look at the reporter and imagine that you are old friends or fellow workers. This may relieve the pressure of trying to sound too professional and prepared. It will also give the interview a real and unrehearsed feeling. This makes you and the information appear more credible. Many more relaxation techniques exist. Find one that works for you and stick with it.

Finally, take comfort in the following facts:

- The media is asking you to do something that you already know how to do . . . talk.
- The media picked you because it feels that you are smart enough to know the answers.
- The media is probably going to ask you about something you just did; thus, recalling a huge number of facts will not be an issue.
- The media wants you because you are not perfect; thus, do not try to be.

Remember that if you make a mistake, the opportunity for a retake may often be given. Speak slowly. People tend to speak faster when they are nervous. Look at the reporter, not the camera. Speak to the reporter as you would to anyone else in a normal conversation.

■ When to Call for Help

Admittedly, there are times when the interview is better left to the department public information officer or the senior officer. These times may or may not be obvious to the rookie EMT, paramedic, or police officer. The following are examples of instances when questions should be referred to a senior officer, qualified person, or public information officer:

- Questions regarding potential investigations.
- Questions regarding department policy.
- Questions regarding current investigations.
- Questions outside of your area of expertise.

- Questions about which you have no information.
- Requests for copies of reports.
- Questions regarding medical information.

Remember that "no comment" is not an appropriate response. Rather, you should simply defer to the appropriate source, senior officer, or public information officer.

Bibliography

1. National Institute of Mental Health, http://www.nimh.nih.gov/anxiety/anxiety.cfm#anx5. November 14, 2003.

2. Narrow WE, Rae DS, Regier DA. NIMH epidemiology note: prevalence of anxiety disorders. One-year prevalence best estimates calculated from ECA and NCS data. Population estimates based on U.S. Census estimated residential population age 18 to 54 on July 1, 1998. Unpublished.

the wrap-up

- You already possess more than the required amount of skill to get through an interview.
- The media is not looking for you to be a polished spokesperson.
- You can have a surprisingly positive impact by admitting to the reporter and to yourself that you are nervous.

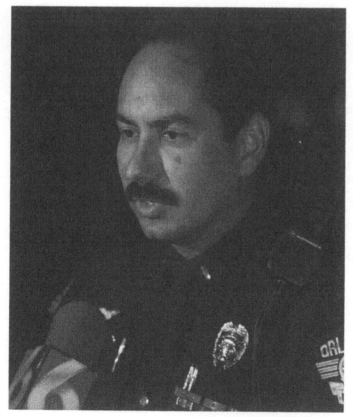

During an interview, speak slowly and look at the reporter, not the camera.

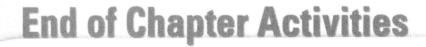

End of Chapter Activities

Review Questions

Read the following questions carefully and answer each question to the best of your ability. Answers can be found in Appendix B.

1. What are some specific phobias?
2. What are some techniques that you can use to combat nerves during an interview?
3. What action should you take if the reporter's questions move into an area where you feel uncomfortable or unqualified?

Scenario Exercise

Carefully read the scenario, then answer the related questions located in the "Your Assignment" section. Check your responses against the answers located in Appendix C.

Scenario

You are the first female fire fighter in a medium-sized fire service. Ever since fire school, the media has pressured you for interviews because you are a woman. You have refused interviews in the past because you felt that you wanted to be treated the same as the others. You have always been camera shy and have disliked being the center of attention. Although you are proud of the career advances and breakthroughs that women have made in the fire service, the thought of an on-camera interview is a nightmare. Your chief has asked you to participate in a media interview that will focus on you as the first woman that the department has hired.

Your Assignment

- What are the conflicting factors in this scenario?
- What should be your response to the chief's request?
- What are some techniques that you can use to relieve your tension?
- What are some interview options that can reduce your apprehension?

The Interview

Learning Objectives

Upon completion of this chapter, you should be able to:

- List the five *W*s and the *H* of an interview.
- Explain the golden rule: "Stay in the box."
- Give examples of "box components" for front-line personnel.
- Give examples of "box components" for a company officer or EMS supervisor.
- Give examples of "box components" for an incident commander or a fire chief.
- Explain how certifications can become problematic at an incident scene.
- Explain why deferring to another source is a good idea.
- List and explain tips for a successful interview.

▥ The Importance of the Interview

"Open mouth and insert foot" is the feeling that many people have when they are asked to participate in an interview. They do not remember the hundreds, perhaps thousands, of successful interviews they have witnessed in their lives. Instead, they remember only the ones in which people have said the wrong thing, have said too much, or have frozen and said nothing at all. They are convinced that they will make some, if not all, of these mistakes during their interview. This chapter explains techniques for surviving the dreaded interview. It also identifies who can say what, provides critical decision paths, and lists techniques for preventing self-induced mistakes.

The interview is the reporter's primary information-gathering tool. Reporters estimate that they gain 75% to 80% of their information through interviews. At a minimum, they want to know who, what, where, when, why, and how. By keeping these five Ws and the H in mind, you can begin to organize information in your mind to prepare for the interview.

Two caveats are worth mentioning before discussing the interview process.

- Any time an interview takes place, the interviewee, or his or her superior, must notify the department's public information officer. This is essential because follow-up with the reporter may be necessary.
- You should never lie to the news media. Besides being unethical, even the best-intentioned lies will inevitably hurt you. If you feel that you have made an error or have misspoken, try to correct the mistake. The media wants truth—not fiction.

These two points are usually included in the department's media policy. Their intent is to ensure effective notice of media contacts and to provide for a possible follow-up with the reporter, if necessary. The honesty component of the second caveat should be self-explanatory. If you lie to the media, the next story on the 6 o'clock news may be this: "An emergency responder has provided false information. What else has he lied about? More about this story at 11 o'clock."

The second component of the second caveat informs emergency responders that if a mistake is made, a chance to correct it will usually be given. Do not try to cover up a mistake or change your story because you may have misspoken. Before you get to that point, however, you must learn to follow the golden rule of media relations.

■ The Golden Rule: "Stay in the Box"

One piece of information to always remember from this book is the Golden Rule of "stay in the box," which refers to you and your role at the emergency scene. Your job function and the things that you directly saw and did define your "box." Staying in the box means that you comment only on things that you have direct knowledge about and that are within your area of responsibility. Do not speculate, predict, or otherwise guess about anything when dealing with the media.

Violation of this seemingly simple concept often gets emergency responders into trouble. A reporter may inadvertently ask you a question that is inappropriate for your level of training, knowledge, or authority. Responding to an inappropriate question is a mistake because the reporter is merely searching for information and you happened to be present.

Failure to follow this simple rule (and ensuing problems from that failure) has soured more than one individual on the motives or morals of the news media. Unfortunately, this blame is often misplaced and could have been avoided entirely if the individual involved had simply "stayed in the box."

As you might imagine, some boxes are larger than others, and they all contain different information. As a rule, individuals with higher status (e.g., officers and supervisors) will have boxes that contain varied and more detailed data.

■ Who Can Say What?

What can be said is determined by your function and direct knowledge of information. Listed below are samples of how these factors dictate what can and cannot be said and by whom.

Operations people such as police officers, EMTs, paramedics, fire fighters, search-and-rescue personnel, lifeguards, or any other individuals who work the front lines of an emergency may have access to the following pertinent information:

- Amount of smoke after arrival
- Intensity of heat
- Number of victims/patients
- Seriousness of injuries (no specifics)
- Location of fire/accident
- Ages of victims/patients
- Special tools that were used in rescue/repair

- Type of watercraft involved
- Breed of dog used in the search
- Hazardous conditions encountered
- Number of emergency personnel on scene
- Exact location of incident

The media will also be interested in technical operations that the general public may have easily observed, but the understanding of which would be enhanced by an explanation from a qualified on-scene professional.

As we proceed up the ladder of responsibility to the level of supervisor and company officer, the amount and quality of information that can be managed increases. These middle-management personnel will be able to address issues that have a greater impact on the incident and those involved. In addition, a company officer, an EMS supervisor, or a middle manager may have access to the following information that would be of interest to the media:

- Time of dispatch/arrival
- Number of gallons needed to extinguish fire
- Plans to evacuate the general public
- Hospital to which patients/victims will be taken
- Outside agencies involved in response
- Tactical plans used, or to be used, in dealing with the situation
- Progress/success of tactical plans
- Estimated time of road/runway/bridge reopening
- Estimated time until utility service is regained

These individuals may also be able to address other areas of the incident, which require more information than those who are assigned specific tasks possess. The next level rung on the ladder of responsibility, and therefore information, would be the highest-ranking official at the scene of the emergency.

An incident commander, the CEO, or the chief will have the authority to address issues at all levels. Although uncommon, they may address operational specifics. More often, they will deal with the most serious problems and may have the following information available (in addition to all information previously mentioned):

- Total resources committed to the emergency
- Number of injuries/deaths involved
- Emergency telephone numbers that the public may call for information
- Existing and future strategies for dealing with the situation
- Expected time frame for the incident to conclude
- Instructions for the public regarding safety

Incident commanders rarely comment on operational specifics but instead deal with the larger impact of the incident and any controversial issues such as death or serious injury to victims or rescuers.

As you can see from these lists, as we progress along the chain of command, the individual's responsibility widens, and the number of people affected by their decisions enlarges. It necessarily follows that comments that the chief or a CEO make will have a wider impact because the subject matter with which he or she deals is broader by nature.

Typically, only an administrator or a government official may overrule the chief, incident commander, or manager. More often, these officials speak only in general terms about the operation and its progress or direction. Their role might include ordering in additional state or federal resources if needed and instilling or restoring public confidence in the overall operation.

The importance of "staying in your box" should be apparent. When a news reporter asks you for a comment on a subject, he or she may have no idea whether you are the best or proper source for this particular piece of information. You may simply be the first person that they encountered at the scene. Just as the incident commander may defer a question on hose line placement to an operations chief, so should a police officer defer questions regarding hospital destination to the paramedic or his supervisor. "Staying in your box" is your life preserver when dealing with the media. Not using it may require you to tread water while surrounded by hungry sharks.

■ Certifications

Many public safety personnel strive to advance their careers and better themselves by obtaining additional certifications. Be proud of your certifications, but also beware. When you are on the scene of an emergency, remember that part of staying in the box is remembering your role at that particular moment. You may hold a fire inspector certification or an arson investigator certification, but none of these should alter or influence your comments to the news media if you are not acting in that capacity at that moment. Consider the following:

- A fire fighter who is reloading hose should not offer opinions about the cause of the fire.
- An EMT applying dressings to a minor bicycle injury should not offer opinions on the mayor's veto of a recent bicycle path tax increase.
- A utility repairperson reconnecting severed gas lines should not offer opinions on the recent increase in utility fees.
- A police officer at the scene of an accidental shooting should not blame politicians for the failure to enact tougher gun laws.
- A lifeguard should not offer suggestions as to which company may have been responsible for the pollution that was recently discovered on the beach.

■ Defer to Another Source

If you get a question that is outside of your expertise, or "official" capacity, simply defer the media to the proper source or to your immediate supervisor. This does not make you look stupid; instead, it shows that you are informed, and it saves the media precious time. Nothing is more annoying to a reporter than wasted time. By sending them to the proper authority, you have increased the reporter's chances of obtaining timely and factual information. He or she may remember you at the next emergency as a valuable source of information and seek your advice. Keep in mind the following when considering whether or not to defer to another source:

- The seemingly simple act of deferring to another source can have a significant impact.
- The reporter will not have to waste time speaking to the wrong individuals.

- Those individuals will not have their duties interrupted.
- Your organization's side of the story will be told.
- The information in the story will likely be more accurate because it came from the most appropriate source.

The simple act of deferring to the appropriate source can greatly influence the flow of information at an emergency scene.

It Is Okay to Say "I Do Not Know"

Do not be afraid to say that you do not know. Not having the information is not a crime. Not knowing does not make you stupid or ill informed. Bluffing, lying, or otherwise providing false or inaccurate information, however, will damage your credibility and the image of your department. Engaging in this type of behavior can even cause you to become the focus of the news story. Reporters are constantly fighting deadlines. If you cannot provide the information that they need, tell them. They will appreciate your respect for their time.

There are many valid reasons for not having the information requested. You could have been assigned to a duty that was nowhere near the incident. You may not be an expert in the subject matter. You should always feel confident that you are making the correct decision by simply saying this: "I do not know."

Tips for a Successful Interview

Now that you understand the importance of the interview for the media, and your role as the public safety personnel being addressed, here are some tips to help you succeed in the interview:

1. **Stay in the box.** As discussed previously, this is your life preserver and source of confidence. You should be able to speak professionally about any topic within your box. A light or buzzer should go off in your head when asked a question that is outside of your box. If this happens, defer the question to a more appropriate source.

2. **Professionalism, professionalism, professionalism.** Acting professional during an interview should be a given. However, because of the nature of our business, we are sometimes vulnerable to being caught in an unfavorable light. Dealing with injury, death, and personal loss can sometimes cause us to lose patience, use inappropriate language, or commit acts that may be viewed as unprofessional.

3. **Listen to the question.** This seems obvious but can sometimes be the cause of a good interview turning ugly. Although we are trained to listen to patient/victim complaints, when we are being interviewed, we may suddenly feel out of our element. If a reporter senses that you are nervous, he or she will often tell you what he or she is going to ask in advance. Slow down. Look at the reporter, and listen to the question. Do not look at the camera, and do not try to hold the microphone. Take a moment to think of what you are going to say and then respond as if you were talking to a close friend. Remember that your interview will be edited after production, and thus, only the important sound bites will be used.

4. **Stay within yourself.** Be yourself and speak in your normal voice. Speak as if you were talking to a friend and avoid the use of jargon. Remember that your message is going to the general public, who may not understand highly technical language.

5. **Do not be afraid to ask to restart the interview.** Everyone, including the reporter, wants the interview to go well. If you misspeak, ask to clarify your statement or restart the interview. Mistakes can be edited after production.

6. **Remember, no one knows your job better than you.** This should give you a great deal of confidence. The reporter is speaking to you because you are the expert in this field. If the reporter already knew the answers, he or she would not need you. Stand tall. Speak slowly. Stay in the box.

7. **Do not touch the equipment.** Nothing irritates videographers more than people who touch their equipment, as these devices often cost more than $20,000. Microphones also seem to say, "Reach out and touch me." You should avoid this instinct, however, because coordinating movement of the microphone is the reporter's responsibility. It can appear more like a wrestling match than an interview when people grapple over control of the microphone.

8. **Do not get confrontational with the media.** If you choose to be interviewed, keep your cool. Sometimes things go poorly, however. If you feel that the interview is rapidly going in the wrong direction, you have some options: (1) Return to the original focus of the interview by restating a previous response. (2) Explain that you do not have information on that topic. (3) Refer back to the question. (4) State that you are uncomfortable and wish to discontinue the interview. If you respond angrily, you can count on that response being the lead story on the evening news. Remember that the media controls what goes on the air, and your performance may become their top story.

Interviewing is more of an art than a science. It is true that the media wants the story, but it also wants you to look good. Your interview will proceed much smoother if you remember these simple rules:

- Never agree to an interview if you feel uncomfortable.
- Never lie.
- Never step outside of your box.

■ Pre-Interview Readiness Checklist

How do you know whether you should participate in an interview? This pre-interview readiness checklist can be used to evaluate whether you are prepared. The novice interviewee or the seasoned professional can use this simple device to help evaluate whether participating in an interview would be a wise decision. If you answer "no" to any of these questions, it may be wise to postpone the interview, as reporters do not want someone on camera, radio, or in print that has nothing to say, is uninformed, or cannot put together a complete sentence.

- Do you want to participate in an interview at this time?
- Do you possess the information that the media is seeking?

- Considering your primary duties, is this the best time for an interview?
- Are you the most appropriate person to comment on the subject matter?
- Can you eliminate the possibility that any comments made now may adversely affect any potential investigation?

the wrap-up

■ The interview is the reporter's primary information-gathering tool.

■ Your job function and the things that you directly saw and did define your "box."

■ Line personnel, supervisors, and top managers all process different levels of information.

■ Nothing is more annoying to a reporter than wasting his or her time.

■ Use language that the general public will understand.

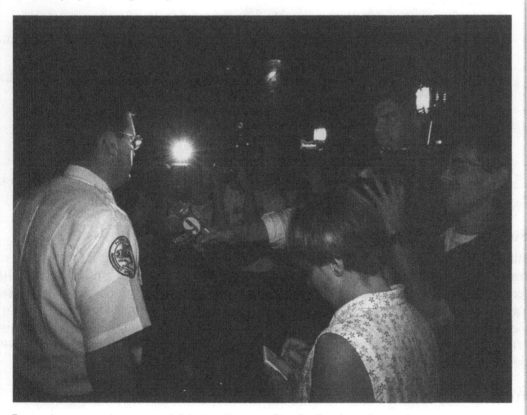

Remember, no one knows your job better than you. Stand tall and stay in your box.

End of Chapter Activities

Read the following questions carefully and answer each question to the best of your ability. Answers can be found in Appendix B.

1. What is the primary tool that reporters use to gather information?
2. What actions should you take if you misspeak or make a mistake during an interview?
3. What is the golden rule?
4. What are some types of information that front-line personnel may disclose to the media?
5. How can additional certifications be a problem at the scene of an emergency?
6. What positive effects can result from simply deferring the reporter to the appropriate source?
7. What are some possible consequences of being confrontational with the media?

(Scenario Exercise)

Carefully read the scenario, then answer the related questions located in the "Your Assignment" section. Check your responses against the answers located in Appendix C.

Scenario

You are with your utility repair crew watching the 6 o'clock news. Earlier in the day you responded to a multiple-car incident with injuries that severed a utility pole at the scene. The media was present but kept approximately 50 feet from the accident scene. You are feeling good about your performance, having re-established service in record time. The news story begins with a close-up of your face and you are heard saying this: "I've seen worse injuries, but not on a babe like this." The reporter goes on to discuss the lack of professionalism that is seen in some who serve the public.

Your Assignment

- How were the comments that you made caught on camera?
- Was the media intruding on your privacy by recording your comments?
- Were your comments appropriate given your role at the incident?
- How might your comments impact public opinion about all public safety providers?
- How might the situation have been better handled?

Traps to Avoid

Learning Objectives

Upon completion of this chapter, you should be able to:

- Explain why only factual information should be conveyed.

- Describe "talking for talking's sake."

- Explain the concept of "hearsay."

- Explain the dangers of speculation.

- Explain the concepts of "off the record" and "not for attribution."

- Explain the concept of "stay on message."

- Explain why jargon should be avoided.

■ Avoiding the Minefields

No one expects you to be a suave and well-spoken media spokesperson. After all, this is not your primary job. Nevertheless, you should want to become as comfortable and professional as possible when being interviewed. One cause of uneasiness is the fear of being tricked or trapped into making a major mistake. Rather than the self-induced errors discussed in Chapter 8, these problems tend to originate from aggressive reporting techniques. All is not lost, however, because these problems can be greatly minimized with proper preparation. This chapter should help you to avoid some of the traps, or minefields, that are associated with being interviewed. Although this information cannot guarantee total success, it can drastically improve your chances of a pleasurable, rather than harrowing, experience.

■ Stick to the Facts

Only the facts of which you have direct knowledge should be discussed with the media. This, of course, excludes any facts pertaining to matters that are currently under investigation and other sensitive issues. If asked for your opinion, beware! Avoid expressing an opinion that the public and others can sometimes interpret as fact. Your position as a professional protector of the public conveys a powerful image. What you say, even if only an opinion, can have a substantial impact. Simply state that you cannot offer a response because of the following reasons:

- The event is still evolving.
- You have no knowledge of that activity.
- You are not qualified in that area.

Your reasons will obviously vary based on the circumstances; however, your rationale should always be truthful and applicable to the situation.

Avoid Talking for Talking's Sake

Be careful not to talk simply for the sake of talking. When questioned during an interview, we somehow believe that we will look smarter if we talk faster and longer. Our desire to speak—sometimes before the reporter has even finished asking the question—must be restrained. If you need a moment to think about your response, take it. If the pause survives the editing process, it may make you look thoughtful and studious. More than likely, they will delete the pause, and you will simply look professional. Remember that you need to control what words come out of your mouth. Take your time, and refrain from being too talkative.

Hearsay

Often a reporter will begin an interview by quoting what another person has allegedly said and will ask for your comment. This is hearsay, which is defined as a rumor or unverified information heard or received from another. It is a dangerous and unprofessional area into which you should never wander. You have no idea whether the person that the media is quoting has actually made the statement. If the alleged statement was never made or someone was misquoted, you may make a bad situation worse by giving continued life to an inaccurate or false story. Never attempt to respond in a situation such as this. Simply state that you cannot comment on what another person may or may not have said. This inability to comment must be distinguished from the refusal to comment. In this situation, you are unable to comment because of the inability to verify the reporter's statement. You are not simply refusing to comment.

Speculation

Occasionally you may be asked to speculate about the outcome of a given situation (a large fire, a multi-vehicle accident, a hazardous material incident, a hostage situation, or an unusually difficult rescue operation, for example). The news media may ask you to comment on the progress of the emergency efforts, second-guess the decisions made up to this point, or predict the outcome.

This sort of speculation is a dangerous form of opinion because it is based on assumptions about the future. If your predictions do not materialize, questions will immediately arise. Was the plan defective? Were the efforts not properly directed? Were the resources insufficient? The possibilities are numerous, and none of them have a positive outcome. Significant energy and resources will now need to be directed toward correcting false assumptions, denying rumors, and setting the facts straight.

If you are asked a question that requires you to predict future events, a statement such as the following would be appropriate: "Everything possible is being done, and we all hope that this incident will have a positive outcome." You should therefore avoid speculation at all costs and save opinions about how you think things should have been done for tactical review at the conclusion of the incident.

Off the Record

Defined as "statements that are not intended to be published," the phrase "off the record" has caused problems for many public safety professionals. Reporters often use off the record comments for background information and to enhance the reporter's understanding of events. Unless you are a seasoned public information officer or media spokesperson, there is *never* any such thing as off the record. Although public information officers and other media liaison people can develop a strong enough relationship with the media to venture into this area, the average emergency responder should avoid off the record comments at all costs. When asked to go off the record, simply state whatever you would feel comfortable stating on the record. As far as you are concerned, on the record and off the record are one and the same.

"Not for attribution" is another term that you may hear. A reporter may agree to not mention your name or attribute the information to you. Instead the phrase, "according to sources" may appear in the broadcast. "Not for attribution" is much like being off the record and should be avoided. Even if your name is not mentioned, the reporter can use your information to investigate the story further.

For example, a reporter can take your information and interview the police chief stating, "Chief, I have been told by sources or by one of your personnel that your response to this call was delayed. Can you comment?" The chief would naturally want to find the source of this information. Leaking information in this manner may not bode well for your career, and you also may have jeopardized an investigation. Remember the golden rule. Be professional and honest.

Stay on Message

Politicians use the "stay on message" technique every day. After a reporter asks a question, the politician responds with a statement that may or may not answer the question. The politician weaves the response into a statement that is important to him or her. If the reporter restates the question, the same process is simply repeated. The reporter may or may not get the answer that he or she needs, but the politician has stated the points that are important to him or her at least once. This is a classic example of staying on message.

After you are called on to take part in an interview pertaining to a certain subject, you begin to formulate responses to possible questions. If, during the course of the interview, you stray into or are led into a different area, you may get that sudden sinking feeling. What happened? How did we get here? What do I do now? The solution is "stay on message." This technique can take practice to appear effortless but can be accomplished if you adhere to some basic rules.

After the reporter poses the question, rephrase and then restate it within your response. This is an example:

"Officer Jones, thank you for agreeing to speak with us today about drunk driving. Officer Jones, do you think your department is doing enough to stop drunk driving?"

Your response: "Thank you for inviting me to talk about our efforts to stop drunk driving. At the ABC Police department, we have devoted significant resources to the prevention of drunk driving through education, as well as the apprehension of those driving while intoxicated."

In this example, you have acknowledged the question and continued on to make your point. This will keep the conversation on subject and help to prevent unexpected questions about more controversial or unexpected subjects.

Given the previous example, what if the reporter were to ask this:

"Officer Jones, you say that your department is devoting significant resources to prevention and apprehension of drunk drivers, yet your department spends more money on squad cars than on drunk driving. How can you justify that?"

You do not want to start a conversation about squad cars. First, acknowledge the question: "Yes, it is true that we spend money on squad cars. They are an important part of our efforts to prevent and apprehend drunk drivers. Without them we would not have been able to apprehend and obtain the convictions of nearly 200 drunk drivers last year." Some people might call this technique "acknowledge and diffuse." You acknowledge the question but weave your response back into your original point. Experienced public information officers have studied this technique and use it effectively during aggressive or controversial interviews.

◾ Jargon

Jargon is specialized vocabulary that is unique to a specific type of work. Most public safety professions are rich in jargon. Although many organizations are making a move to a "plain text" type of language, especially in radio communications, our professions still contain many words and phrases that are unique to our work. Unfortunately, when we use these words and phrases during an interview, we can alienate and confuse the public. An experienced reporter will always ask you to explain any terms that are too technical for the general public to understand. Taking the time to do so takes away from the story. If the entire interview ends up with you explaining every word you utter, the interview will virtually be unusable to the media.

Whenever making a statement to the media, do the following:

- Speak as if you were addressing someone who is not in your profession.
- Imagine that this individual has little or no understanding of your work, but do not speak down to them.
- Speak simply and clearly.

◾ Other Terms to Avoid

Along with jargon, certain terms should never be used. Some of these are listed here as a reminder to always be professional. The following terms, although not all-inclusive, should never be used when speaking with the media:

- Terms that are demeaning to any particular sex.
- Terms that are demeaning to any race.
- Terms that are demeaning to any religious group.

* Terms that are demeaning to any age group.
* Terms that are demeaning to individuals with a physical or mental disability.
* Terms that are demeaning to individuals with any particular body size or type.
* Terms that are demeaning to any individuals in any particular vocation.

the wrap-up

- Only the facts of which you have direct knowledge should be discussed.
- Do not comment on what another person may or may not have said.
- Avoid speculation at all costs.
- When asked to go "off the record," simply state whatever you would feel comfortable stating "on the record."
- Stay on message and stay out of trouble.
- Avoid jargon.

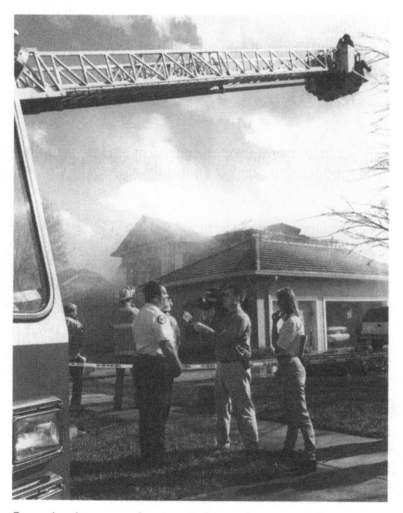

Remember that you need to control what words you speak. Take your time and refrain from talking for talking's sake.

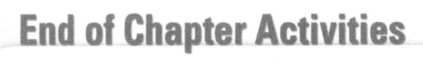

End of Chapter Activities

Review Questions

Read the following questions carefully and answer each question to the best of your ability. Answers can be found in Appendix B.

1. What are some reasons why you may not have the facts that the media requested?
2. What is the definition of hearsay?
3. What is one way that reporters may make use of "off the record" comments?
4. What is the definition of "off the record?"
5. What is the difference between "off the record" and "not for attribution?"
6. What problems may result from supplying information "off the record" or on a "not for attribution" basis?
7. What technique may be useful during aggressive reporting?

Scenario Exercise

Carefully read the scenario, then answer the related questions located in the "Your Assignment" section. Check your responses against the answers located in Appendix C.

Scenario

A 6-year-old child is trapped inside a storm water drain. The rescue is particularly difficult and has been going on for hours. Tension is high, and everyone, including the child's parents and emergency personnel, is exhausted. Several media outlets are present. While inventorying equipment for the next stage of the rescue, you are approached by a reporter. He asks his cameraperson to stand back and give you a few moments alone so that he can talk to you. As he hands you a cup of coffee he asks your opinion on how the rescue is progressing. He also asks "off the record" about the little girl's chances of making it out alive. Finally, he wants to know whether the delays in getting specialized equipment at the scene may have lessened the girl's chances.

Your Assignment

- Because the cameraperson was asked to stand back, what assumptions can you make?
- What dangers exist in expressing your opinion regarding the progress of the rescue?
- What should your response be to his request for an "off the record" statement?
- Why is it impossible and inadvisable to answer his last question?

Role Reversal

Learning Objectives

Upon completion of this chapter, you should be able to:

- List several types of proactive media events.
- Explain the benefits of these types of activities.
- Explain the role of the media in catastrophic events and public notification.
- Explain the role of the public information officer in marketing.

■ Why Would You Ever Want to Contact the News Media?

You want me to call the news media? There are many instances when you can and should contact the media. One benefit to this proactive approach is the professional relationship that will develop over time.

Most circumstances in which you contact the media will be attempts to highlight your agency or department. Although you may not get the coverage that you desire because of more pressing stories, you should try. This is not the time to air dirty laundry, such as the implementation of a new disciplinary policy. In most cases, it is unwise to contact the media to cover what is destined to be a negative event. Exceptions to this rule exist, however. In cases in which an employee's actions have already drawn a great deal of public interest, such as an arrest, you may want to be proactive to demonstrate your willingness to cooperate with the media and the public. This does not mean using the employee as a sacrificial lamb, but rather providing a public statement of the known facts and a promise to keep the media and the public updated. Because it takes about ten good press stories to offset one bad one, the message is clear: Grab all of the good press that you can get! This chapter addresses the many mutual benefits of a professional relationship with the media.

Open Houses

Open houses are excellent opportunities for you to showcase your facilities. Remember that your position and department are more than likely supported by a customer tax base. Your customers' only contact with you may be at a time of crisis. By working with the media to publicize your organization, the public gets an opportunity to see what its tax dollars are purchasing. It is an invaluable public relations opportunity that should not be missed.

Promotions, Education, and Certifications

Departmental promotions are an excellent opportunity to highlight your personnel. Although new ambulances, fire trucks, police cruisers, and other equipment are exciting, personnel are the backbone of what we do. It is important that the community sees that your personnel are working hard to advance within the organization. Your customers will appreciate the fact that they have career-minded individuals serving the community. It is astonishing how underused this form of free press is in our profession. We never hesitate to call the media to view a new helicopter but seem to forget to announce the latest promotion or college degree obtained.

Certifications may also merit a call to the media. When our personnel are recognized for this achievement, it is a good opportunity to tie the certification to the specific activity. For example, diving certifications can be displayed with the involved equipment. In the case of high-angle rescue certifications, a demonstration can be staged in which the students must rappel down a tower to receive their certification. Police drug-detection dogs and their handlers can be showcased in conjunction with recently obtained training certificates or confiscated drugs.

Training Drills

The electronic media, especially the television sector, tends to love training drills because of the strong visual content. Television is all about images, and training sessions are an excellent opportunity to show that you have the right stuff. New trucks, large streams of water under pressure, people climbing 100-foot ladders, new drug-detection dogs, and other possible images are sure to be a hit with the media and the public.

The equipment and training used during these drills undoubtedly cost a great deal of money. Be sure to invite the taxpayers to view the demonstration, which will inevitably draw more media attention because of the easy and immediate public reaction. Are you trying to get your story across? Are you hoping to impress the public? Are you hoping to temporarily tip the scales in your favor to counteract an inevitable bad story? Of course!

Hazardous Material Situations, Contaminations, and Product Tampering

Occasionally, you will need to respond to a hazardous material situation. Even if you do not handle the situation yourself and must call in a specialty unit from a neighboring community, the media can be very valuable in notifying the community at large of the danger. Large toxic gas clouds may require residents to move to a shelter. The radio and television media represent the best method of notifying residents of an emergency. This action can inform the residents and prevent panic. Contaminated water can affect thousands of people over a brief period. Door-to-door notification is not feasible. The media is your only option in this emergency.

Product contamination on a large scale is not an impossible terrorist target. Any product that is consumed in large quantities poses a potential risk. If such an attack were to happen, the media is the only practical way to notify the large numbers of potential consumers.

Announcements of missing persons, escaped prisoners, and other important community news are additional areas where the media can be a valuable ally. Do not be afraid to enlist the media in your efforts to serve and protect the public.

Weather-Related Natural Disasters, Evacuations, and Road Closings

Floods, hurricanes, mudslides, tornadoes, tidal surges, and extreme heat or cold are all situations in which the media can work with you to preserve life and protect property. By issuing warnings about these conditions, you can mitigate damage and prevent injuries and casualties. This is a truly valuable opportunity for you and the news media to make a positive impact on the safety of your community.

Many of the previously mentioned situations could precipitate an evacuation within your community. Hazardous materials spills can be managed by moving people to a shelter, but they sometimes necessitate evacuation. Imminent dangerous weather conditions can also prompt evacuations. By removing people from the danger before it arrives, you and the media are preventing injury and possibly death in your community.

Announcing road closings are another way that the media can help provide a public service. Roads can be closed for a multitude of reasons. Traffic delays can cause a disruption of medical as well as fire and law enforcement service to your community. By working with the media to announce these situations, you can prevent traffic delays and thereby keep travel routes open for emergency.

■ The Public Information Officer and Marketing

As a public information officer, or someone assigned media relations duties, you must be able to market your organization. Although some consider our services essential, no service can escape the inevitable budget cut at some point. You must continually market your services to the media, as well as to the general public. Marketing to the general public is generally covered under the events listed previously here (open houses, equipment displays, for example). Other public marketing options can include the following:

- Public education efforts, such as CPR and first aid classes
- Safety checks, such as car seat installation
- A program to host children's birthday parties for a minimal fee (developed by an enterprising department)
- A written column in the local newspaper that provides tips on fire safety, crime prevention, or seasonal events, such as water conservation or Christmas tree safety

Marketing to the media begins with marketing yourself. Your efforts could include the following:

- Planning visits to the offices of the media outlets in your area (be sure to call ahead for an appointment)
- Taking and distributing any preprinted information you may have describing your organization
- Leaving your business card and asking for theirs
- Asking for a tour of the facility and taking pictures for your newsletter or annual report

- Inviting media representatives to speak at public information office association gatherings
- Planning joint projects, such as educational videos

the wrap-up

- Grab all of the good press you can get!
- It is important that your community sees that your personnel are working hard to advance within the organization.
- Strong visual images are sure to be a hit with the media and the public.
- The media can be very valuable in notifying the community of any type of danger.
- If marketing is part of your job, be proactive and creative.

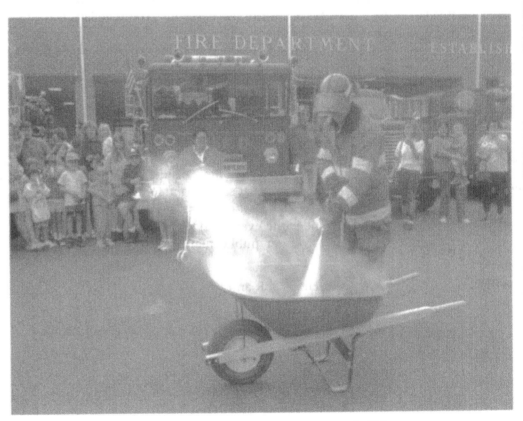

Open houses are excellent opportunities for you to showcase your facilities.

End of Chapter Activities

Read the following questions carefully and answer each question to the best of your ability. Answers can be found in Appendix B.

1. What types of events should represent the majority of the instances in which you contact the media?
2. What effect can open houses have on your local taxpayers?
3. Which opportunity is most suited to the television media?
4. Which media type is best suited for notifying residents of a toxic waste spill?
5. What part can the media play during weather emergencies?

Scenario Exercise

Carefully read the scenario, then answer the related questions located in the "Your Assignment" section. Check your responses against the answers located in Appendix C.

Scenario

Your chief e-mailed everyone in the department asking for volunteers for three upcoming television interviews. The topics to be covered are new equipment, training, and new taxes to pay for your services.

Your Assignment

- Explain which interview would be more suited for a rookie employee and why.
- Explain which interview would be more suited for a veteran employee and why.
- Explain which interview would be more suited for the public information officer and why.

High-Profile Incidents

■ Testing Your Metal

High-profile incidents are defined as any incident that stresses the resources of an agency beyond its day-to-day capabilities and results in elevated levels of concern in the organization and the community. At one time, we rarely thought of or prepared for these incidents. Today, however, high-profile incidents are not as rare and are not unique to large agencies. With the threat of terrorism rising worldwide, an isolated water supply that has been infected with a biological toxin can easily generate the same high media inquiry as a bombing in a crowded mall. This chapter addresses this new phenomenon and provides some guidance to assist you in minimizing its associated problems.

■ Causes

Although the causes of such incidents can vary, the resulting strain placed on the organization will be similar. Examples of these causes include airplane crashes, major fires in high-rise buildings, acts of terrorism, public health epidemics, organizational scandals, acts of war, or other mass casualty situations. The fact that so many different events can have the same effect justifies our preparation for such incidents. Some of these events, especially terrorism, are the result of a rapidly changing world. Protecting the people that we serve means that we must now prepare our personnel for the media response to these events.

Organizational Impact

Although the credo of "stay in the box" serves as an effective life preserver in high-profile situations, additional information can be beneficial. It is important to realize that this is not a typical event. Acknowledging this circumstance is the first step in protecting yourself and your organization. This should provide you with a heightened awareness and will hopefully cause you to be more critical in your decision making.

You should not let the magnitude of the event distract you from getting your job done. Remember Fundamental Truth #1: Your primary responsibility is your job. It is easy to be distracted and say or do something that is atypical in high-stress situations. Your judgment may be affected by the following factors if you are not prepared:

- Individuals may be assigned a duty that is unfamiliar.
- Work hours may be lengthened.
- Needed materials may be unavailable or slow to arrive.
- Families and the media may pressure you for results.

Although the public information officer will be very useful in events such as these, every member of the organization needs to remain focused and professional.

Hidden Challenges

Incidents that span longer time frames often come with unique media-relations challenges. One such challenge, which can surface and involves emergency responders, is the "idle time interview." Reporters will conduct this seemingly harmless interview during down time at high-profile incidents. Emergency workers are frequently tired or bored and must be particularly careful about the content of any statements made under these circumstances. Any of these factors can lead to erroneous or even inflammatory statements. Your casual comments may be viewed or heard by loved ones of victims and the public. Any negative comments that you make can be viewed as poor performance by emergency workers, or a prediction of a poor outcome. These statements can have a devastating effect. On the other hand, light-hearted comments may be viewed as a lack of concern or true commitment to the disaster and may have the same negative effect.

The extended time frame that is often associated with such incidents can lead to other challenges as well. Because the outcome of the particular event is yet undetermined, the media will often begin searching for background stories. You may be awakened at your home after an exhausting 12-hour shift to find a reporter with cameraperson in tow standing at your front door. These "people stories" often focus on the emotional impact of the event on emergency workers and families of victims. You would certainly have justification in a case like this to decline the interview. This refusal is certainly not the same as a "no comment" response and needs to be differentiated as such.

If, however, you decide to grant the interview, you need to proceed with caution. If, at any time, the interview direction changes and you become uncomfortable, stop the interview and ask that the reporter return to the original topic or simply end the interview. Although you may be tempted to speak more freely during these off-duty home interviews, remember that to the public you are always viewed as being on duty, no matter where you are.

Say what you know and what you did and refer any off topic or matters in which you lack the proper knowledge or experience to the proper source.

■ Role of the Media at High-Profile Incidents

Any high-profile incident will generate media interest. If the incident involves an immediate threat to pubic health or safety, the media may fill a public notification role. If the incident involves fraud or other violation of public trust, the media may fill a public advocate role. If the incident involves political issues, the media may fill a governmental watchdog role. Indeed, the media may, and most likely will, mold itself to investigate more fully and relay the information concerning any significant news event. Remember that what you do as public safety personnel represents a significant event and generates news coverage.

The role of the news media at a high-profile incident will therefore be forged by the incident itself and may change as events unfold. It is best to remember that the media's basic function is to report news—any news. Its role and your interaction with the media at high-profile incidents will not change significantly, except in the following ways:

- The media will be competing with more news agencies for the same information.
- More media means a greater chance that you will be interviewed.
- The added pressure of the event may cloud your judgment.
- The public information officer, if available, should coordinate most of the interviews.
- You have a greater chance of being asked inflammatory or controversial questions.

Some individuals might propose that isolating the media in these events solves these challenges. As you should have learned by reading the text and solving the chapter problems and scenario exercises, neither isolating the media nor adopting a "no comment" stance is an acceptable approach to interacting with the media. Isolating the media will only force them to sources that may be inaccurate or unsympathetic to your efforts. A more effective and sound approach to managing the information highway during such incidents is to:

- Stay in the box.
- Utilize available resources, such as the public information officer.
- Stick to your department's media relations policy.

the wrap-up

- The role of the news media at a high-profile incident will be forged by the incident itself and may change as events unfold.
- A heightened awareness should cause you to be more critical in your decision making.
- Incidents that span longer time frames often come with unique media-relations challenges.
- Don't forget to stay in the box.
- Make use of the available resources , such as the public information officer, and your department's media relations policy.

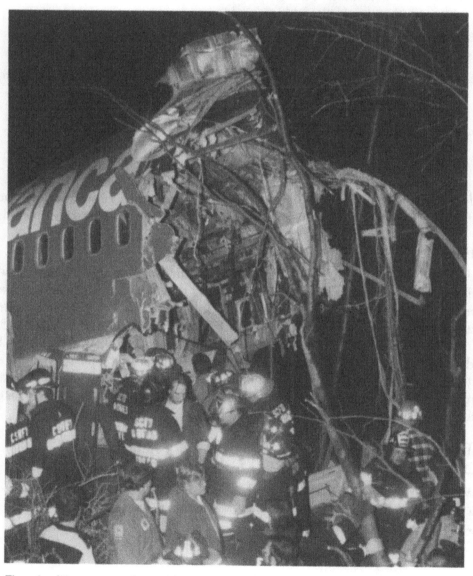

The role of the news media at a high-profile incident may change as events unfold.

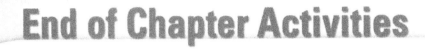

End of Chapter Activities

Review Questions

Read the following questions carefully and answer each question to the best of your ability. Answers can be found in Appendix B.

1. What is the definition of a high-profile incident?
2. What are three examples of high-profile incidents?
3. What factors can make the idle time interview problematic?
4. Is isolation of the media an option at these incidents?
5. What is one way the role of the media at a high-profile incident may differ from a typical emergency response?

Scenario Exercise

Carefully read the scenario, then answer the related questions located in the "Your Assignment" section. Check your responses against the answers located in Appendix C.

Scenario

You and your colleagues are watching a television news account of an interview with an emergency responder at the scene of a building that is being evacuated because of a biohazard terrorist scare. The individual being interviewed seems to be uncomfortable and anxious. As the interview progresses, it is clear that the interviewee is not happy with the direction in which the interview is proceeding or with the questions being asked. At one point, a verbal argument breaks out between the reporter and the emergency responder. After that point, the tone of the interview changes from covering an emergency response to a terrorist act to the effects of the pressure felt by emergency responders in responding to incidents such as this.

Your Assignment

- What explanation could there be for the tension between the reporter and the emergency worker?
- What questions could have prompted the argument?
- How might the general public view any inappropriate comments made by either party?
- How might the situation have been better handled?

Post-Test

1. The Freedom of Information Act (FOIA) protects:
   a. Medical records
   b. Criminal records
   c. Federal records
   d. All of the above

2. A reporter's requirement to inform you that he or she is a member of the media is based on:
   a. Federal law
   b. Executive order
   c. State law
   d. None of the above

3. Which form of news draws the most media attention?
   a. Good news
   b. Bad news
   c. Ugly news
   d. All of the above

4. Television media often considers video footage to be:
   a. A small part of the story
   b. The entire story
   c. A minimal part of the story
   d. None of the above

5. In a high-profile incident, national media representatives should:
   a. Be given preferential treatment
   b. Be shunned in favor of the local media
   c. Be treated the same as other media representatives
   d. None of the above

6. "No comment" is an appropriate response:
   a. When there are fatalities involved
   b. When you do not like the reporter
   c. When the reporter asks an inappropriate question
   d. None of the above

7. Making the statement "no comment" can cause people to think that:
   a. You are being uncooperative
   b. You are uninformed
   c. You are hiding something
   d. All of the above

8. Public speaking should be a mandatory part of every public safety provider's responsibilities.
   a. True
   b. False

9. A police officer is asked for his or her opinion on the outcome of a hostage situation. He should:
   a. Keep comments brief

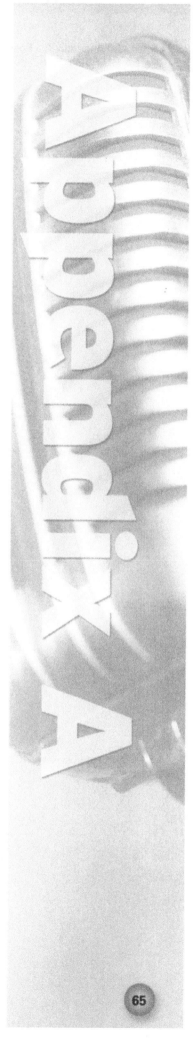

b. Supply only factual information

c. Never speculate

d. All of the above

10. Saying that you do not have the information that the reporter is seeking is:
a. Never appropriate
b. The same as saying "no comment"
c. An acceptable response
d. None of the above

11. Off-the-record comments are:
a. Never appropriate for front-line personnel
b. Only allowed when you trust the reporter
c. Proper under emergency circumstances
d. None of the above

12. Instances when you should call the media include:
a. When new employees are hired
b. When hazardous material spills on a major highway
c. When new equipment is purchased
d. All of the above

13. A heightened sense of awareness is important in what type of events?
a. Events involving routine matters
b. Annual events
c. High-profile events
d. Political events

14. Factors that increase stress at high-profile events and may lead to misquotes include:
a. Long work hours
b. Unavailable or late arriving resources
c. Unfamiliar assignments
d. All of the above

15. What role might the media play if a high-profile incident involves fraud or other violations of public trust?
a. A criminal investigation role
b. A political advisor role
c. An inside informant role
d. A public advocate role

Post-Test Answer Key

1.	c	6.	d	11.	a
2.	d	7.	d	12.	d
3.	c	8.	b	13.	c
4.	d	9.	d	14.	d
5.	c	10.	c	15.	d

Chapter Review Answers

Chapter 1

1. Technology is, and will continue to be, the single most influential factor in the amount of media interaction that we receive.
2. Advertisers, who are interested in the number of viewers, are the primary source of revenue for the media.
3. The media has reduced in-house operations costs by using more wire copy, local or freelance photographers, file footage, and large video news services such as Reuters and the Associated Press.
4. The media gathers information, prepares stories, and makes broadcasts that inform us about local, state, national, and international events. It presents points of view on current issues and reports on the actions of public officials, corporate executives, special-interest groups, and others in positions of power.
5. Your department's media policy, your position within the organization, and your first-hand knowledge of the information requested should govern your interaction with the media.

Chapter 2

1. Patient age, gender, and hospital destination are usually released to the media.
2. The First Amendment of the Constitution guarantees freedom of the press.
3. Ethics can be defined as "the system of morals of a particular person, religion, or group."
4. The media does not have the right to enter private property to take photographs or for any other reason without the permission of the property owner.
5. The FOIA applies to federal records within an agency.
6. HIPAA regulates protection of patient information.
7. A retraction may result in more attention being given to a sensitive situation and further investigation.

Chapter 3

1. News can be defined as new information, information previously unknown, or recent happenings.
2. Good news would include items such as public CPR classes, open houses, promotions, new equipment, and rescued animals.
3. Simple fires, auto accidents, burglaries, downed utility lines, assaults, and other routine emergency responses would be considered bad news.
4. Ugly news can include major fires that get out of control, arrests of department personnel, charges of misconduct, inappropriate public statements, and failed rescue attempts.
5. Human factors often make the ugly type of news the most covered by the media.

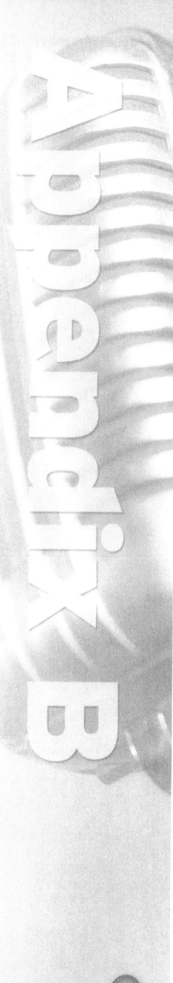

Chapter 4

1. The print media uses the written word to convey their message.
2. The television media considers video to be the main part of the story; it often is the story, simply surrounded by commentary.
3. Images can be recorded from hundreds of feet away. Helicopter-mounted and mobile microwave truck-mounted cameras can record images from even greater distances.
4. Always assume that the microphone is recording and that the camera is live.

Chapter 5

1. A media policy provides two key tools to assist you in communicating with the media. Those tools are direction and baseline performance objectives.
2. The purpose of a departmental media policy is to provide guidelines for the release of public (not confidential or private) information to print and electronic news media.
3. The policy should be written so that it conveys a message of **full** and **impartial** cooperation with authorized news media representatives.
4. As a general rule, the media may photograph anything in public view.
5. Regular briefings may keep freelancing and speculation to a minimum.

Chapter 6

1. A "no comment" policy will only serve to alienate the media and the public.
2. Having your spokesperson tell your side of the story insures that the message is factual and consistent.
3. "No comment" conjures up images of alleged criminals seated in a courtroom.
4. Saying that you do not know or that you do not have time to answer at the moment are acceptable alternatives to "no comment."
5. Some legitimate reasons for not wanting to participate in an interview include:
   * You are afraid or uncomfortable with the entire interview process.
   * You may not have the skills necessary to participate.
   * You may not want to be the center of attention.
   * You may be afraid to say the "wrong thing."
   * You may have had a bad experience with the media in the past.

Chapter 7

1. Common specific phobias include fear of closed-in places, heights, escalators, tunnels, highway driving, water, flying, dogs, and injuries involving blood.
2. The best technique for combating fear of public speaking is practice. Other techniques include admitting your nervousness to the reporter, taking slow, deep breaths, and giving the interview with a buddy.
3. Defer questions that make you feel uncomfortable or that you do not feel qualified to answer to another more qualified source.

Chapter 8

1. Reporters estimate that they gain 75% to 80% of their information through interviews.

2. If you feel you have made an honest error or have misspoken, say so and correct the mistake.

3. The golden rule of "stay in the box" refers to remembering your role at the emergency scene. Your job function and the things that you directly saw and did define your "box."

4. Front-line personnel may release information such as: the amount of smoke after arrival, the intensity of heat, the number of victims/patients, the seriousness of injuries (though no specifics), the location of the fire/accident, the ages of victims/patients, special tools used in rescue/repair, hazardous conditions encountered, the number of emergency personnel on scene, and the location of the incident.

5. None of your certifications should alter or influence your comments to the news media if you are not acting in that capacity at that moment.

6. Deferring the reporter to the appropriate source can have the following benefits:
   • The reporter will not waste time speaking to the wrong individuals.
   • Those individuals will not have their duties interrupted.
   • Your organization's side of the story will be told.
   • The information in the story will likely be more accurate because it comes from the most appropriate source.

7. You could become the lead story. You will also present a less than favorable image for your profession. Remember, the media controls what appears on the air or in print.

Chapter 9

1. You may not have the information requested for one or more of the following reasons:
   • The event is still evolving.
   • You have no knowledge of that activity.
   • You are not qualified in that area.

2. Hearsay is defined as a rumor or unverified information heard or received from another.

3. Reporters often use "off the record" comments for background information, perhaps to enhance the reporter's understanding of events.

4. "Off the record" can be defined as a statement that is not intended to be published.

5. "Not for attribution" means that a reporter may agree not to mention your name or attribute the information to you. Instead of your name, "according to sources" may appear in the news story.

6. Even if your name is not mentioned, the reporter can use your information to investigate the story further. It may not bode well for your career if you are discovered to be that source.

7. "Stay on message" can be used in aggressive interviews. It allows you to diffuse the situation and stay on topic.

Chapter 10

1. Most of the instances in which you contact the media should be attempts to positively promote your agency or department.
2. Open houses allow the public an opportunity to see what their tax dollars are purchasing.
3. The electronic media, especially television, will love these opportunities because of the strong visual content.
4. The radio and television media represent the best method for notifying residents of an emergency.
5. By issuing warnings about adverse weather conditions, the media can mitigate damage and possibly prevent injuries and death.

Chapter 11

1. A high-profile incident can be defined as any incident that stresses the resources of an agency beyond its day-to-day capabilities and results in elevated levels of concern in the organization and the community.
2. Examples of high-profile incidents include airplane crashes, major fires in high-rise buildings, acts of terrorism, public health epidemics, organizational scandals, acts of war, or other mass casualty situations.
3. Boredom, weariness, and a desire to return to the action are three factors that can make idle time interviews problematic.
4. Isolating the media will only force them to talk to sources that may be inaccurate or unsympathetic to your efforts.
5. The role of the media and your interaction with them at high-profile incidents will not change significantly, except for the following elements:
   - Local media outlets will be competing with more news agencies for the same information.
   - More media means a greater chance that you will be interviewed.
   - The added pressure of the event may cloud your judgment.
   - The public information officer, if available, should coordinate most of the interviews.
   - You have a greater chance of being asked inflammatory or controversial questions.

Scenario Answer Summaries

Chapter 1

You were proud of your newly certified dog's performance. Unfortunately, you let your enthusiasm blind you to the sensitive nature of the situation. An acceptable response would have been "yes." No more and no less information is necessary. Identifying the body is the job of law enforcement. Your "box," or role, which you performed well, was to locate the victim. Let the specialists handle the identification. Do not speculate. Because the general public perceives you as an expert, the family may take your tentative identification of the body as fact. Your credibility will be ruined if Mrs. Cramer shows up at a neighbor's house 2 hours after your interview hits the air.

Chapter 2

You made a comment regarding the mayor's health. This was not only unprofessional but in violation of many regulations regarding protection of patient privacy. You have speculated on the possible causes of the patient's illness. Your comments fueled public speculation that the mayor may be unfit for office. You assumed that your casual conversation was "off the record," undoubtedly based on your previous relationship with the reporter. It is essential to separate personal relationships from professional responsibilities.

Chapter 3

This scenario is a prime example of "ugly" news. Although full disclosure of available information should take place, this is not your function, and the following answers should address the concerns of the scenario. This question can be answered with a simple response of "I do not have that information, but I can refer you to someone who might." Litigation against the department is not your specialty, and these types of questions should be referred to your superior, the public information officer, or the chief. It may be prudent to deflect the question with a response of "I do not see what relevance that would have to this tragic incident. I do know that the department is attempting to provide any assistance possible to all parties involved, including the two officers who were also injured in the performance of their duty."

If you are unaware of any statements that they are alleged to have made, say so. If you are aware of their statements, say so, but add that you are sorry for the family's loss and concerned for the recovery of the two officers. Acknowledging the statement but not commenting on it is an effective way to avoid controversy.

If you know the policy, share it with the reporter. It is a matter of public record, and the reporter will obtain it eventually. If you feel uncomfortable with the interview, defer the question to your superior or the public information officer. Your department may face several disadvantages in this situation. By not having a full-time public information officer, you may not be able to quickly refer the reporter to someone who may have the answer they seek. You are not the public information officer and should not make an official statement. A press release should be generated. The press release will remove the suspicion that your department was hiding something or "protecting its own" with preferential treatment.

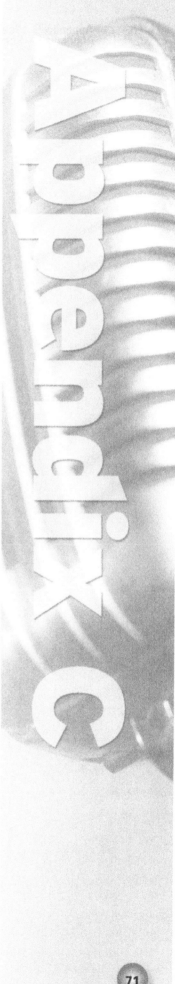

Chapter 4

As a public safety provider, you may get frustrated when safety concerns are not quickly addressed. You may have personally responded to some of these accidents and may have commented out of frustration about the apparent delay in placing a traffic signal at this location.

If you were asked to comment on the need for a traffic light at that intersection, you should have restricted your comments to specific accidents that you have responded to at this intersection. The town may actually be in the process of studying the intersection for the addition of a signal. Not being aware of this could make your comments seem unprofessional and inappropriate. As a law enforcement professional, any negative comments that you make could be construed as a failure of town officials to appropriately address this situation.

Misquotes do occur. If you feel that you were misquoted, you and your department need to determine whether a retraction or correction is worthwhile. If you were not misquoted, then you need to analyze what you may have said to the media.

You must remember that as an emergency responder your opinion on safety issues carries substantial weight in the eyes of the public. Your comments could set off a negative public reaction that is unwarranted and unnecessary.

Chapter 5

You should always remember that your job is your first priority. If talking to the media in any way interferes with your treatment of the girl or protecting the many other swimmers present, simply state that you cannot speak with them at this time because of your other duties.

By attending to your job and contacting your supervisor, you have set the wheels in motion for the proper and professional response to this situation. Officials should immediately recognize the seriousness of this incident and respond accordingly. This response should include an official press release.

The two factors that make this story newsworthy are (1) a young child was involved and (2) the mother is making accusatory statements.

Someone who is not a lifeguard is credited with the rescue of the child. A good public information officer will seize this opportunity to promote water safety, give credit to the young rescuer, and reinforce the fact that children should always be supervised.

A media policy would give you a course of action and guidelines as to what can and cannot be discussed.

The mother's comments should be taken with the proverbial "grain of salt," as she is emotional because of her child's accident. If you avoid getting defensive and provide support to her and her child, you are avoiding a no-win situation and may be laying the groundwork for a positive public relations opportunity in the future (such as hosting a "Water Safety Awareness Day," with the little girl as the guest of honor).

Chapter 6

As both incident commander and operations officer at this incident, you have your hands full. Although your frustration level may be high because of the suspicion of arson, you are not the fire marshal or a member of the arson investigation squad. Your comments should be limited to operational questions, with all other questions referred to the appropriate people.

If you suggest that the owner has committed arson, you may be guilty of slander. Even if you are not accused, you have engaged in unprofessional speculation. As suggested previously, your comments should be limited to operational specifics. Even if you are certified in the area of arson investigation, your role at that moment was operations.

Chapter 7

Your sense of pride for women's career advances and your overwhelming dislike of being interviewed on camera are at odds in this scenario. You are undoubtedly feeling additional pressure because of the chief's request that you take part in the interview and your rookie status in the department.

Honesty about your feelings toward interviews should be expressed clearly to the chief. He or she does not want you pressured into something and does not want a poor interview about his or her department.

Along with the tension-busting techniques that are mentioned in the chapter, the buddy interview might be particularly useful in this situation. Having a classmate or coworker stand alongside you will help to bolster your confidence and divert some of the attention from you.

Chapter 8

Today's cameras and microphones are incredibly sensitive. Fifty feet is easily within the distance to record images and audio. Any comments that you may have made were likely recorded. As a public safety provider, anything you do or say in the public domain is fair game for the media. You were on a public street and therefore should have been much more professional in your comments. The comments were inappropriate and unprofessional.

Will the public assume that all utility workers behave in this manner? How might this impact the next request for a tax increase for increased utility services? How might this impact the next case in which one of your coworkers is accused of inappropriate sexual behavior? Issues such as these can impact you and your organization for years and cost thousands of dollars to resolve. Proper management of this situation would have simply been to be professional in the performance of your duties and to always assume that you are being recorded when the media is present.

Chapter 9

Do not assume anything, except perhaps that you are being recorded. Just because the cameraperson is standing back does not mean that you are not being recorded. We have already learned that cameras can record from great distances.

Although you are certainly entitled to your opinion, this is not the place to express it. Remember that you are considered the expert. Everyone who hears your statement, including the girl's family, will consider it to be fact. A general statement such as this can generally be considered safe in these situations: "We are doing everything that we can, and we hope that she will be all right."

Remember, never go "off the record." Your response should be the same on or off the record. Stick to the facts and do not create false hope.

You may or may not know whether there was a delay in receiving any specialized equipment. If there is someone in charge of that equipment, refer the reporter to that person or to the public information officer. Do not speculate, do not predict, and do not attempt to answer questions that you are not qualified to answer.

Chapter 10

Training is probably the best interview situation for the rookie. Training is something that applies to everyone, and a rookie would be most familiar with new training advances. This should be a low-pressure and easy interview.

New equipment is an interview for the veteran. A veteran will have perspective and be able to provide comparisons between new and existing (Hint: Do not say "old.") equipment. They will be knowledgeable and make the department look professional.

New taxes are definitely an area that is better left to the public information officer. This sensitive area will require a fine balance between additional costs to the customer and valuable services provided. Sensitive subjects such as this should always be left to the professionals.

Chapter 11

Incidents with weapons of mass destruction are becoming more of a possibility. Responding to an emergency in which you have little experience is always more stressful. A weapon of mass destruction incident has the potential to affect emergency personnel for years to come.

The interviewee also seemed uncomfortable with the questions being asked. If the questions are making you uncomfortable because they are outside of your realm of knowledge, refer the reporter to the proper person. If the questions cannot be answered because of a lack of information, ask for time to acquire the needed data. If the questions are inappropriate or confrontational, ask that the interview be stopped. No further explanation is necessary because the interview was voluntary and was subject to your full and willing participation.

This is a no-win situation for the interviewee and his department. The public will see one of the people entrusted with their safety as out of control and argumentative. Never argue with reporters. Confrontations with reporters will frequently pull the focus of the story away from the incident itself.

This situation should have never occurred for several reasons. The interviewee was obviously uncomfortable and should not have done the interview. This was an extremely high-stress incident, and personnel may have needed more time to diffuse before speaking in public. Use of a public information officer or an official who was not directly exposed to the potential threat may have been a better choice for an interview in this case.

Sample Media Policy

Subject:	Any County Sheriff's Office General Order	Number:
Public Information Procedure		
Effective Date:		Revision:
September 1, 2002		**November 1, 2003**
Amends:	Anytown, USA	Rescinds:
Related References:		Accreditation Standards:
Reviewed By: Date:	Reviewed By: Date:	Reviewed By: Date:

I. **PURPOSE**: The purpose is to facilitate methods and procedures for the dissemination of information to the media and the public.

II. **POLICY**: It is the policy of the _____ County Sheriff's Office to reasonably accommodate the news media and the community by providing information in a timely and accurate manner that is not otherwise exempt or confidential.

III. **PROCEDURE**: Within established guidelines and procedures, the sheriff's office shall notify, in a timely, fair, and impartial manner, members of the media on matters of public interest. Such notification will not be made during such time that notice would compromise the integrity of any ongoing criminal investigation or agency operation. In such cases, media notification will be made as soon as possible.

IV. **RESPONSIBILITY**:

A. Management Responsibility

1. Supplying public information and communicating are direct responsibilities of management personnel. These responsibilities may be delegated operationally. When practical, an immediate supervisor or designated media liaison officer (MLO) should respond after being fully informed by knowledgeable participants. At no time will members of the sheriff's office intentionally mislead or misinform members of the media.

2. The ranking sheriff's office member present at a disaster or crime scene or the agency media liaison officer, if requested by the ranking agency member, is responsible for providing relevant, timely, and accurate information to the news media.

3. Routine media inquiries will be handled by the MLO but may be handled by the watch commander when the MLO is temporarily unavailable. When the MLO is not available (vacation, illness, etc.), the sheriff will designate a backup person to act in that capacity.

B. Personnel

1. Sheriff's office personnel shall take into consideration the deadline time of the respective news media representative(s) when he or she requests information regarding a sheriff's office–related incident and will oblige the representative as much as possible in meeting this deadline. This pertains particularly to supervisors, records, and the MLO.

2. The MLO should be notified as soon as possible so that he or she can respond and deal with the media at the scene or relay information to them via the telephone.

3. Members shall not seek publicity through the news media or furnish information to them for the express purpose of seeking personal notoriety while acting in an official capacity for the sheriff's office.

V. **NEWS RELEASES AND FLASH REPORTS:**

A. Flash reports and news releases shall be used to provide all local media (print and television), as well as other media outside of the local area, with information related to major incidents. The frequency with which flash reports and news releases are issued will depend on the types of activity occurring each day.

B. The MLO or his or her designee will disseminate news releases and flash reports. Copies of the flash report should be given to the front desk supervisor in charge and the MLO.

C. The MLO or designated supervisor will initiate/distribute flash reports in an expedient manner on major incidents.

1. During the MLO's normal working hours, the on-duty watch commander or his or her designee will notify the

MLO in a timely manner of any major incident(s) occurring on his or her shift and give a synopsis of such incident(s).

2. When the MLO is unavailable, the on-duty watch commander will respond to news media representatives' requests for information, if this information can be handled in a timely and reasonable manner. If the information requested needs extensive research before responding, the on-duty watch commander will either take the request for information and forward the request to the MLO or he or she will refer the media representative to the MLO; this information will be handled during the MLO's normal working hours.

D. Supervisory personnel will notify the MLO of the following major incidents:

1. Homicides, kidnapping, and/or robbery of financial institutions or other significant robberies

2. Natural or man-made disasters resulting in a loss of life and/or extensive property damage, as well as major commercial fires and explosions

3. Aircraft accidents, traffic accidents with fatalities, and school bus accidents involving any injuries investigated by the SSO

4. Bombs or incidents in which a device is found or a major evacuation occurs within SSO jurisdiction

5. Missing persons under 12 years of age, missing persons when foul play is suspected, manhunts when an extensive search is involved

6. Raids, demonstrations, strikes, or disorders involving groups of people

7. Shootings/stabbings by citizens or law enforcement officers

8. Deaths by other than natural causes (i.e., fire, electrocution, and drowning)

VI. **CONSISTENCY**: Members of this agency will strive for consistency in releasing information to the media for public dissemination. Information that is normally released should not be withheld based solely on a decision relating to the personal prominence of those involved. Conversely, information generally not routinely distributed should not be put forth solely as a result of personal prominence.

VII. **VICTIM CONSIDERATION**: Victims should be informed that this state's Public Records Law requires that information regarding complaints and criminal investigations be released to the public when such cases are completed unless specifically exempt or made confidential by law. Consideration should be given to victims' requests for no publicity or no public disclosure of a crime to which they are a party. However, no employee will guarantee to any victim or reporting party that a reported case will not receive publicity.

   The decision not to release information or documentation about a particular crime or incident or the name of a victim or reporting party must be made by the bureau commander or designee in conjunction with the Office of the General Counsel. This decision will be made only after due consideration is given to whether such release would endanger an ongoing investigation and is consistent with this state's Public Records Law.

VIII. **GUIDELINES FOR THE RELEASE OF INFORMATION**:

   A. Ongoing Investigations

      1. The sheriff's office is not required to release active criminal investigative or intelligence information that is exempt or confidential related to ongoing investigations. Information made confidential by law shall not be released to the media or public except as authorized by law. Exempt information related to an ongoing investigation may be released if the sheriff deems the release of the information necessary for law enforcement purposes. Employees shall not provide the media or the public their opinions of the guilt or innocence of the accused or the merits of the case.

         a. Information related to the prior criminal records, character, or reputation of the accused may be released with the discretion of the sheriff.

         b. Agency photographs of an arrested person may be released, providing that it will not jeopardize the investigation.

         c. The existence of a confession, admission of guilt, or statements or refusal of statements made by the accused may be released with the discretion of the sheriff.

d. The results of any examinations or tests of the accused may be released with the discretion of the sheriff.

e. The identity, testimony, or credibility of any witness may be released under the discretion of the sheriff.

f. Personal information pertaining to the victim shall be released in accordance with this state's Public Records Law (i.e., personal information pertaining to victims of sexual battery shall not be disclosed or released).

g. Information pertaining to juveniles shall be released in accordance with this state's Public Records Law and other relevant laws.

h. Information received from other agencies shall not be released without concurrence of that agency. When the sheriff's office is involved with other agencies during incidents or matters of mutual responsibility and concern, sheriff's office personnel will cooperate and coordinate fully with those agencies in public information. Generally, the agency or primary jurisdiction should make appropriate news releases citing assisting or secondary agencies. At any time that other agencies assist this agency in an operation or investigation, the assistance will be noted in any news release.

2. Certain information is always open for inspection and release:

a. Date, time, location, and nature of crime reported

b. Name, gender, age, and address of person arrested (except for certain juveniles)

c. Name, gender, age, and address of victim (except victims of sex offenses/child abuse)

d. Date, time, and location of incident and arrest

e. Crime charged

f. Documents required to be given to arrestee for discovery in criminal cases (the court can prohibit release before trial if that release would be defamatory to the name of the victim or witness OR jeopardize safety of victim or witness AND impair the ability of the state attorney to locate/prosecute codefendant)

g. Information and indictments (except persons not in custody/under arrest)

IX. ACCESS TO CRIME SCENES:

A. Generally, whether a crime scene or a scene of another nature, police have an obligation to preserve the integrity of the scene to gather evidence and for other necessary police activities.

   1. Law enforcement personnel will delineate the specific crime scene area and prevent all persons from entering that area for such a length of time as there is a need to do so.

   2. The general public may be excluded from not only the crime scene itself, but also from a reasonable area around the crime scene for crime scene preservation purposes and to control general access to the area.

   3. However, officers must recognize the need for news media representatives to fulfill their obligation to view the immediate crime scene area for newsgathering or photographing purposes. News representatives will be accommodated, so far as conditions permit, to go as near as practicable to the crime scene itself. News representatives are not to be considered the same as the general public in the area of a crime scene, but rather as persons to be accommodated so that they may fulfill their responsibilities.

B. If a law enforcement–related incident is within a private building or dwelling, police personnel will secure and protect the building area as may be necessary in order to protect the crime scene. Under such circumstances, all persons may be excluded from the crime scene area until processing is accomplished.

   1. If a news media representative makes a request to enter a building or part thereof and such entry is not precluded because of police related purposes, the news representative must obtain permission from the owner or other person in charge of the building or dwelling.

   2. If permission is not given and so stated to the news representative in the presence of law enforcement personnel, the media shall not enter the private dwelling.

C. At fire-related incidents, the decision to allow properly identified reporters and photographers to pass beyond fire lines or restrict them from a fire area will be the responsibility of the on-scene fire commander.

D. Photography

1. Photographing of any individual in custody may not be authorized within the confines of the sheriff's office buildings. Photographing of prisoners outside of the building is permitted; however, prisoners will not pose for photographers. Photographing of uncovered bodies will be done at the discretion of the news media, who will assume full responsibility for any such photographs or film.

2. Photographing sheriff's office–related incidents, including motor vehicle accidents, accident injuries, and uncovered bodies, will be at the discretion of the news media, provided that the process does not interfere with rescue personnel or the investigation.

X.   PERSONS RESPONSIBLE FOR THE RELEASE OF INFORMATION:

A. The MLO or shift supervisor will be responsible for coordinating and releasing information pertaining to crime incidents and operational activities for the agency.

B. Statements of policy expressing official positions of the agency responses to criticism of the agency, statements pertaining to pending or ongoing civil litigation involving the agency, disciplinary matters, personnel, policies, internal affairs, and officer-involved shootings shall be made only by the sheriff, the MLO, or designated person.

C. Occasionally it might be required that media personnel obtain information directly from a particular bureau. This information is often generic to the bureau. In the event that information is released and time permits, it is the responsibility of a supervisor in that bureau to advise the MLO of its intent along with the content of the interview. This is done to insure that the MLO is continually kept informed of what information is being disseminated to the media.

D. Agency members are not required to honor any news media request involving sheriff's office–related incidents while off duty. In the event the member chooses not to answer off-duty inquiries, the media representative will be referred to either the MLO or the on-duty watch commander.

XI. SOURCES OF INFORMATION FOR THE MEDIA:

A. In order to facilitate the dissemination of crime/incident information, news media representatives should pursue the following channels for information:

1. The MLO is to be contacted in person or by telephone for the desired information during normal working hours, Monday through Friday. The MLO will notify the media on issues, press releases, and scheduled press conferences. It will be the responsibility of the MLO or a designee to assist the news media at all press conferences.

2. Media representatives requesting feature story interviews with on duty members of the agency should first contact the MLO (excluding on the scene) and explain the request. If such interview is granted, the member shall give out information in accordance with this general order.

3. All personnel should understand that it is standard media policy that any and all conversation with a representative of the news media is on the record and is subject to being quoted.

4. After the MLO's normal working hours, the media representatives may call the on-duty watch commander to obtain a synopsis of a major incident that may have occurred on the shift.

XII. INDEX:
Flash Reports,
Release
Information,
Classified
Media Liaison Officer
Press Release
Public Information Procedure

I have read and understand this order.

Sample Press Release

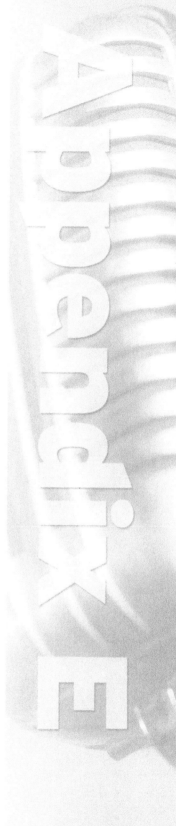

For Immediate Release

Name of Organization _____

Address _____

Topic/headline _____

1st paragraph (should include most important information)

2nd paragraph (next most important information)

3rd paragraph, if necessary (least important information)

Prepared by _____

Name of author _____

Title _____

Contact numbers _____

Date _____

Time _____

    More (to indicate the second page)

or

    # # # (to indicate the end of the document)

Glossary

Anchor: The coordinator or chief reporter of a newscast.

Associated Press wire: A not-for-profit news cooperative that is owned by 1,550 U.S. daily newspaper members who elect a board of directors to manage the cooperative. In the United States alone, the Associated Press serves 1,550 newspapers and 5,000 radio and television stations. In addition, it has more than 8,500 newspaper, radio, and television subscribers in 112 countries.

Beat reporter: A reporter who is assigned to cover news in a specific area (e.g., police, fire, local government, local industry).

Broadcast/electronic media: Organizations involved in radio, television, or Internet-based news services.

Commentator: One who reports and analyzes news events.

Deadline: A time limit imposed on the reporter before which the story must be presented.

EMT: An individual who is trained to assist victims of medical, traumatic, or environmental emergencies through the use of noninvasive techniques.

File footage: Video footage previously recorded and stored for future possible use.

Fire fighter: An individual trained to assist victims of fire and other emergency situations, in addition to the preservation of property through fire prevention and extinguishments.

Freedom of Information Act (FOIA): A federal law that allows access to certain types of records when proper application has been made.

Freelancer: A reporter or photographer who is paid on a piecemeal basis by various news organizations.

Hazardous situation: Conditions that require specialized equipment or procedures because of their chemical and/or biological makeup.

Health Insurance Portability and Accountability Act (HIPAA): Government guidelines mandating individuals or organizations that maintain or transmit health information to establish or maintain appropriate administrative, technical, and physical safeguards to ensure the integrity, confidentiality, and availability of the information collected.

Idle time interview: An interview that the media uses to fill news gaps or to add background information to an event that spans a greater than usual timeframe.

Jargon: Specialized vocabulary that is unique to a specific type of work.

Libel: Any written or printed matter tending to unjustly injure a person's reputation.

Live feed: A real-time transmission of a news story from a remote location.

Microphone: A device used to convert sound into an electronic signal for transmission to another location.

Microwave: An electromagnetic wave used to transmit signals from a remote location to a news studio for broadcast.

Natural disaster: An event originating from meteorologic or other natural causes that has a substantial negative impact on people and/or property.

News: New information, information previously unknown, or recent happenings.

News release: A prepared statement, usually written, that presents facts regarding a specific incident or event. It provides the "who, what, where, when, and why" of the event, in addition to a person to contact for further information.

Paramedic: An individual trained to assist victims of medical, traumatic, or environmental emergencies through the use of invasive techniques.

Phobia: An irrational, excessive, and persistent fear of some thing or situation.

Press conference: A structured event held to make announcements, ask for assistance, or otherwise inform the general public about an event or issue.

Print media: News outlets that distribute information through the written word via newspapers, magazines, etc.

Privacy Act: Protects personal privacy by limiting disclosure of records without prior written consent from the subject of the record in question.

Public information: Information regarding policy, events, or procedures involving an organization. This may include any newsworthy information that is not legally protected, does not interfere with department operation, does not infringe on the rights of individuals, or does not endanger departmental personnel.

Public information officer: An individual selected to serve as the central source of information to be released to the media and the public at large.

Quote: The repetition of a passage or statement.

Reporter: An individual who gathers and/or presents information for a media source.

Reuters: A 150-year-old newsgathering and reporting company that packages and transmits text, video, news photography, and graphics to print and broadcast media, Web sites, and wireless services on six continents.

Satellite truck: A vehicle that relays remote broadcasts via orbiting satellite to a studio for rebroadcast.

Slander: The utterance of a falsehood that damages another's reputation.

Stringer: A part-time local correspondent for print or electronic media outlets.

Video camera: A device used to record video and sound images.

Wire copy: News reports that are broadcast by large newsgathering organizations such as Reuters (sometimes rebroadcast by smaller television, radio, and print markets).

Additional Credits

Chapter Opener Art

© Ablestock

Chapter 1

Page 6 © Craig Jackson/In the Dark Photography

Chapter 2

Page 15 © Spencer Grant/Photoedit

Chapter 3

Page 19 © Robert E. Klein/AP Photo

Chapter 4

Page 23 © Curt Hudson/AP Photo

Chapter 6

Page 34 © Julia Malakie/AP Photo

Chapter 7

Page 39 © Craig Jackson/In the Dark Photography

Chapter 8

Page 47 © Craig Jackson/In the Dark Photography

Chapter 9

Page 53 © Craig Jackson/In the Dark Photography

Chapter 10

Page 58 © Michael Heller/911 Pictures

Chapter 11

Page 63 © Steve Spak/911 Pictures

Notes

Notes

Notes